STO

616.(
GREEl
DR. G   WHAT   RY
MAN SHOULD KNOW ABOUT HIS
PROSTATE

D1550340

DO NOT REMOVE
CARDS FROM POCKET

ALLEN COUNTY PUBLIC LIBRARY

FORT WAYNE, INDIANA 46802

You may return this book to any agency, branch,
or bookmobile of the Allen County Public Library.

Dr. Greenberger's
WHAT EVERY MAN
SHOULD KNOW ABOUT
HIS
— PROSTATE —

also by Mary-Ellen Siegel

Her Way (1976)

Chemotherapy: Your Weapon Against Cancer
(1978)
(co-author: Ezra M. Greenspan, M.D.)

What Every Man Should Know About His Prostate
(1983)
(co-author: Monroe E. Greenberger, M.D.)

More Than a Friend: Dogs with a Purpose (1984)
(co-author: Hermine M. Koplin)

Her Way: Second Edition (1984)

Reversing Hair Loss (1985)

The Cancer Patient's Handbook (1986)

The Nanny Connection (1987)
(co-author: O. Robin Sweet)

Finger Tips (1988)
(co-author: Elisa Ferri)

Dr. Greenberger's

WHAT EVERY MAN
SHOULD KNOW ABOUT
HIS
—— PROSTATE ——

Revised Edition
by Mary-Ellen Siegel, M.S.W.

Senior Teaching Associate
Department of Community Medicine (Social Work)
Mount Sinai School of Medicine
City University of New York

Foreword by Michael E. Gribetz, M.D.

Assistant Clinical Professor of Urology
Mount Sinai School of Medicine
City University of New York

WALKER AND COMPANY, NEW YORK

Allen County Public Library
Ft. Wayne, Indiana

Copyright © 1988 by Mary-Ellen Siegel

All rights reserved. No part of this book may be
reproduced or transmitted in any form or by any means,
electronic or mechanical, including photocopying,
recording, or by any information storage and retrieval
system, without permission in writing from the Publisher.

First published in the United States of America in 1988
by the Walker Publishing Company, Inc.

Published simultaneously in Canada by Thomas Allen & Son
Canada, Limited, Markham, Ontario.

Library of Congress Cataloging-in-Publication Data

Greenberger, Monroe E.
   Dr. Greenberger's what every man should know about
his prostate.

   Rev. ed. of: What every man should know about his
prostate. 1983.
   Bibliography: p.
   Includes index.
   1. Prostate—Diseases—Popular works. I. Siegel,
Mary-Ellen. II. Greenberger, Monroe E. What every
man should know about his prostate. III. Title.
RC899.G73   1988   616.6'5   88-10763
ISBN 0-8027-1023-9

Printed in the United States of America

10 9 8 7 6 5 4 3 2 1

In loving memory of my father
Monroe E. Greenberger, M.D.
1896–1982
and my uncle
Arthur J. Greenberger, M.D.
1891–1964
They were brothers, friends and urological associates for forty-four years, and were teachers to generations of urologists and physicians to thousands of appreciative patients.

CONTENTS

FOREWORD

Having known Monroe Greenberger as an esteemed colleague and (in his later years) as a patient, I was honored and flattered when Mary-Ellen asked me to write the forward for the second edition of this manual.

The book stands as a memorial to a great man and a superb clinician—humane, compassionate, and astute, always bringing to his patients a combination of experience and tradition coupled with an academician's and scientist's need to remain current and innovative. In this revised edition, considerable effort has been made to keep the reader current on the state of the art and yet preserve the warm insightful approach to patients that defined Monroe Greenberger as a great urologist. Many of the anecdotes from Dr. Greenberger's clinical practice provide us with a view of his common-sense wisdom—the human touch that should be a dominant attribute of any clinician.

What Every Man Should Know About His Prostate is not a textbook but rather a manual to guide the patient/consumer in seeking and evaluating help. As our population matures and ages, more and more men reach the "prostate" age. Understanding the diseases that afflict the prostate will enable the patient to know when to seek help and to understand the advice given him by his physician. A knowledgeable and well-informed patient and his family are partners in care with the physician and form a team working toward better health.

As one reads the various chapters, one should avoid the pitfall of self-diagnosis. Symptoms of many conditions overlap, and symptoms alone do not provide a reliable basis for diagnosing the cause of a patient's complaint.

Mary-Ellen Siegel has written a sensitive and thoughtful manual dealing with a wide range of topics affecting our maturing population. Benign prostatic hypertrophy, prostatitis, carcinoma of the prostate, incontinence, and sexual dysfunction are conditions that are often diagnosed, but they are poorly understood by the lay public. This manual will provide the patient with the background to understand his body better and to participate knowledgeably in his own health care.

MICHAEL E. GRIBETZ, M.D.
Assistant Clinical Professor of Urology
Mount Sinai School of Medicine
New York

ACKNOWLEDGMENTS

Many people gave of their time and expertise to help bring the original edition of *What Every Man Should Know About His Prostate* to you. They included: Claire Bennett, M.S.W. Herbert Brendler, M.D., Irving M. Bush, M.D., Gail Button, R.N., Michael Carrera, Ph.D., William Fair, M.D., William Gersh, M.D., Deborah Green, M.S.W., Ezra M. Greenspan, M.D., Michael E. Gribetz, M.D., George Klein, M.D., Elliot Leiter, Gonzalo Lopez, M.D., Karen Martin, M.A., Arnold Melman, M.D., George Nagamatsu, M.D., Helen Rehr, D.S.W., Gary Rosenberg, Ph.D., Hans E. Schapira, M.D., Sidney M. Silverstone, M.D., Norman Simon, M.D., Judy Spielberg, R.N., Moses Swick, M.D., and Joseph Trunfio, M.D.

A number of people were especially helpful to me in preparing this revised edition. They include: Gail Button, R.N., Eleanor Driscoll, I. Del Carmen-Weill, R.N., J. Lester Gabrilove, M.D., Howard Goldman, M.D., Louis Lapid, M.D., Alfred Rosenbaum, M.D. all of the Mount Sinai Medical Center in New York.

Irving Bush, M.D. and William Fair, M.D. again were helpful, as was Morton Goldfarb, M.D., and Sol Usher, M.D. Eleanor "Kay" Workman was extremely supportive and helped provide needed information and insights into the Greenberger office practices.

Special thanks to Charles Gerras, Richard Winslow, Nancy Green, Mary Horan, and Steven Gray.

A very special note of appreciation to Michael Droller, M.D. Chairman of the Department of Urology, Mount Sinai School of Medicine.

Michael E. Gribetz, M.D. Assistant Clinical Professor, Department of Urology, Mount Sinai School of Medicine, New York gave enormously of his time and expertise—again above and beyond all expectations. He was indispensable, and I am enormously grateful to him.

INTRODUCTION

The original edition of *What Every Man Should Know About His Prostate* developed through the collaborative efforts of my father, Monroe E. Greenberger, M.D., and me. We spent many weekends with a tape recorder, as I asked questions and Dad answered them. Until everything a man (and a woman who cares about him) should know about his prostate was clear to me, we did not stop! Mother would make us break for lunch, and then we would be back again at work. When Mother died, we put the manuscript away; but we took it out again in the summer of 1982, to revise and polish it.

When the first draft of the revised manuscript was completed, my father suggested that we ask Michael Gribetz, M.D.—an Assistant Clinical Professor of Urology at the Mount Sinai School of Medicine—to look it over. Dr. Gribetz made many suggestions, so we felt assured that the final text of the book reflected current practices as well as the long experience of my father. We acknowledged and thanked Dr. Gribetz for "his time and expertise above and beyond all expectations."

A few weeks after Dad had approved of the illustrations and we had sent the galleys off to friends and colleagues for prepublication comments, he had a stroke and died. He had practiced urology until the very end; and in his eighty-six years, he had lived a full and happy life.

As I began the job of revising the book, I called upon Dr. Gribetz again. We spent several hours discussing current findings and practices in urology, even before I sat down at my word processor to begin work. In addition, I spent many hours in the medical library at the Mount Sinai School of Medicine, reviewing the latest studies on the prostate. Eleanor "Kay" Workman, who managed my father's office for forty years, was a great source of information about Greenberger office practices and was an enthusiastic supporter of this revised edition. Today she works for another urologist, Sol Usher, M.D.

Since the earlier edition there have been important advances in the diagnosis and treatment of prostate disorders—particularly cancer of the prostate. Ultrasound—which allows the physician to see the size of the prostate with greater clarity than earlier studies—new blood tests, and new office biopsies mean that prostate problems can be treated earlier than ever. At one time surgery for cancer of the prostate usually rendered a man impotent; because of new nerve-sparing surgery, this is no longer so.

All of these new findings are included in this edition of the book. When the first draft of the manuscript was completed, Dr. Gribetz carefully reviewed it, making suggestions and corrections, and he then reviewed later drafts. It is with special pleasure that I thank this very fine urologist for having helped to update this revised edition of *What Every Man Should Know About His Prostate*.

I know my father would be pleased.

MARY-ELLEN SIEGEL, M.S.W.
Fresh Meadows, New York
August, 1988.

A NOTE TO THE READER

The author and publishers have exerted every effort to ensure that information set forth in this book is in accord with common practices. However, in view of ongoing research and differences of opinions, some practices may vary and may change.

No part of this book is intended to provide personal medical care to any individual and we urge you to consult your own physician on all matters relating to your health.

1

THE PROSTATE

When several urologists get together to discuss prostate problems, they usually agree that treating these problems constitutes a major part of their office practice. Of course, each man's prostate condition seems special to him, but the variations in this area are in fact remarkably few. An expert can treat most prostate ailments effectively, with a minimum of discomfort for the patient.

Preventing prostate disorders, however, is another matter. The incidence of such disorders increases every year. Curiously, this increase is a direct result of the medical successes that prolong life, because the longer a man lives, the more likely he is to experience prostate trouble. According to some estimates, half of all men need to consult a physician about prostate discomfort at some time during their lives. Men who live to the age of eighty almost invariably suffer, or have suffered, from some type of prostate disorder.

Although the causes of prostate trouble vary greatly, the most common symptoms (which remain strikingly similar) are all too familiar to many men:

- Frequent or urgent need to urinate, including during the night
- Hesitancy in beginning to urinate
- Discomfort or pain during urination
- Inability to maintain the usual urinary stream

- Pain in the pelvic or rectal area
- Sensation of incomplete emptying of the bladder

Other problems may also signal prostate trouble. Among these are the following:

- Diminution of caliber and force of the urinary stream
- Inability to stop urinating abruptly; instead, continuing to dribble
- Blood in urine
- Nausea, dizziness, or unusual sleepiness—sometimes the result of "silent prostatism," in which prostatic obstruction exists but there are no symptoms, yet adversely affects renal function.

Most of these symptoms are very annoying and can interfere with certain life-styles. A truck driver, or a salesman who travels around town or has a long commute to work each day, will find the frequent need to urinate intolerable. But a man who has a bathroom near his office and who is seldom away from such a convenience for more than an hour or so may tend to ignore these symptoms. Similarly, a person who needs to get up often at night but easily falls back to sleep may not be too troubled, either.

If the symptoms have developed gradually over a period of time, a person may hardly be aware of them. Alternatively, he may think that it is normal at his age to have such problems. But it is not normal; and if ignored, it can get worse and become that much harder to treat.

One symptom—blood in the urine—must *never* be ignored. Any time a man voids some blood (even if he feels no pain) there is reason for concern. The blood might be visible only at the beginning of the stream; it might color the entire stream; or it might just be noticed at the completion of urination. In each case, it indicates something important. A urinalysis should be sought promptly from the individual's personal physician. Although blood in the urine may be the result of something other than a urological problem, it generally does show that something is wrong in the genitourinary tract or kidneys. Blood in the urine may be caused by anything from a simple inflammation to a stone or tumor. Painful hematuria (blood in the urine accompanied by pain during urination) suggests a stone in the urinary tract or a urinary tract infection, and of course requires prompt medical attention.

It is important to realize that one or more of these symptoms may be a sign of other disorders, as well. For this reason, a man should resist the temptation to diagnose his own ailment. Instead, he should approach his personal physician, who can do the preliminary examination and (if necessary) refer him to a urologist for a further evaluation.

THE NORMAL STATE

Most people have some basic knowledge about the prostate. They know, for instance, that it can interfere with urination and that it has something to do with a man's sex life (although rather indirectly)—but that's usually the extent of their knowledge. But there is much more to learn and understand. If all men (and women, too!) were better informed about the prostate, they would recognize when something goes wrong, and they could prevent minor problems from becoming major ones. Informed patients work well with physicians in making decisions that influence their physical and emotional future.

The prostate, exclusively a male property, is located

next to the inner wall of the rectum, directly below the bladder (the elastic sac that stores urine, which is formed in kidneys) and around the urethra (the tube that carries urine from the bladder through the body and out through the penis). It is usually described as a musculoglandular structure consisting of two major components: an internal zone, and an external zone. Its surface can easily be felt by the physician when he performs a rectal examination. Unfortunately a man cannot perform regular self-examinations (as women are advised to perform on their breasts), unless he's a contortionist.

In its normal state, the prostate is about the size of a chestnut, but it is shaped somewhat like a pyramid. Just as men vary in height and weight, so their organs vary in size, but generally the normal prostate is about 1½ to 2 inches wide at its widest and weighs about 15 to 20 grams (less than 0.75 ounce).

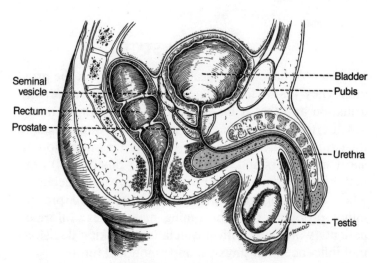

THE GENITOURINARY SYSTEM

The prostate is often likened to an apple with the core removed. The urethra passes through the prostate, as the core would pass through an apple. Naturally, if the prostate becomes swollen (as a result of infection or some disease), it will crowd the urethra and cause discomfort.

The prostate starts to develop in the twelfth week of embryonic life. It is tiny in a newborn boy but can be felt by the pediatrician upon careful examination; it doesn't increase in size until puberty. At puberty the prostate begins to grow to its normal mature size—stimulated, it is believed, by the increase in male hormones. Its size then remains constant until a man nears fifty, when the gland again begins to enlarge. The reason for this second period of growth at this time of life has not been established with any certainty, but it has been commonly attributed to a combination of aging and possibly a change in male hormones. Whatever the cause, it is unfortunate that this change in prostate size occurs at roughly the same age when many (but not all) men may be experiencing a change or decline in sexual performance. It is also a time when a man may begin to have doubts about his ability to advance farther in his career; his children may be growing away from the family; and his wife may be experiencing an uncomfortable menopause or developing new career interests outside the home. Thus this period may be difficult for him in many ways, and symptoms of prostate enlargement (better known as *benign prostatic hypertrophy,* or *BPH*) only tend to exacerbate these concerns.

It is not at all uncommon for men to live into their seventies, eighties, and nineties without major medical problems; but because an estimated 60 percent of men over the age of sixty have some symptomatic prostatic enlargement, and up to 95 percent of eighty-year-old men have such a condition, doctors see more and more such patients. Cancer of the prostate is also on the rise, because it usually attacks older men. Autopsies performed on elderly men whose cause of death is unrelated to cancer of the prostate add substance to the suspicion that cancer of the prostate is almost universal in men over eighty; but because of its slow progress and the absence of overt symptoms, it is frequently not recognized. Infections, inflammations, and congestion are prostate problems that continue to affect males of all ages.

THE GENITOURINARY SYSTEM

The prostate gland, a compact organ, is surrounded by a dense and fibrous "surgical" capsule. When a man says that he has had his prostate removed because it became enlarged, it is most likely that the gland (including most or all of the enlargement) has been removed from the capsule. Only in very special situations—such as when the operation is to treat cancer of the prostate—does a urologist remove the capsule as well as the gland.

This relatively tiny gland, which is capable of causing so much trouble, has only one known function: to contribute to and activate the production of a fluid that transports sperm cells during ejaculation. The prostate secretes $\frac{1}{10}$ to $\frac{2}{5}$ teaspoon of prostatic fluid daily; this amount increases to $\frac{1}{2}$ to 4 teaspoons of fluid when sexual arousal occurs. At the junction of the bladder and prostate lies a sphincter that prevents semen from flowing backward into the bladder at the time of ejaculation. The prostate may have other functions, but they are not yet fully understood or defined. The prostate does produce enzymes, and perhaps hormones, too; whether these enzymes and hormones perform any necessary function or contribute in any way to a man's general health has not been established.

A man whose prostate gland has been removed is almost never able to impregnate a woman, even though sexual intercourse is normal for him in every other way. This may be due in part to the absence of prostatic fluid and in part to the surgical procedure, which involves widening the bladder neck and usually leads to a reversal of the sperm's normal route, sending it back into the bladder. This procedure should not, however, be depended on for contraception.

In all males, sperm travels a rather circuitous journey. It is produced in the testicles and takes approximately ten weeks to mature. At that time, sperm leaves the testicles and enters the epididymides (singular, *epididymis*), where it is stored for another three weeks. The epididymis is a tubular structure behind each testicle. After the sperm has matured, it travels through the vas deferens—a tube or duct attached to the epididymis. The two vasa deferentia (one from each testicle) loop behind the bladder, ending at points called *ampullae*. The sperm is stored in the ampullae until released through ejaculation. Next to the ampullae are the seminal vesicles; these saclike glands secrete a nutrient fluid that helps sustain the sperm. Connected to the seminal vesicles are ejaculatory ducts, which run through the prostate gland. The sperm and seminal vesicle fluid flow through these ducts, picking up nutritious fluid from the prostate, as well as fluid from the Cowper's glands (two pea-sized glands on either side of the urethra). This fluid then passes through the urethra and is expelled through the penis at time of ejaculation.

SOURCES OF PROSTATE TROUBLE

Much of what we know about the prostate has come to light since the end of the nineteenth century. The anatomy and physiology of the prostate gland were first understood at that time, and scientists realized that the prostate could become a site for cancer. As many as 4,000 years ago, however, the Egyptians treated the symptoms resulting from prostatic disease and abnormal growth. Even then they knew that a man who had to struggle to urinate (or was unable to urinate at all) not only experienced great pain, but was also in danger of death. They inserted reeds or copper or silver tubes through the penis and urethra to widen the urinary passageway and allow urine to escape. This procedure often turned out to be a lifesaver.

When urine is backed up in the bladder, crystallization often takes place and stones are formed. In ancient times, these stones were removed with the same crude instruments used to widen constricted urethras. The medicine men who performed the procedures later became known as lithologists (from the Greek word *lithos,* meaning stone). Not until much later was the prostate itself recognized as the source of the problems.

Among the many problems a man can have with his prostate are infection, congestion, and BPH (enlargement). Infections are often caused by bacteria that may have traveled from nearby or even from a distant site such as teeth, sinuses, or tonsils; they may also be the result of a past instance of venereal disease. Congestion can develop from various causes, including (according to many practicing urologists) even a simple change in sexual habits. BPH usually occurs some time after the age of fifty. Although all of these problems may produce similar symptoms, a treatment that is appropriate for one may be radically wrong for another.

8

Cancer of the prostate is more serious than any other prostate problem, but early detection and prompt treatment can be successful. Cancer of the prostate often can be diagnosed before any symptoms are obvious; for that reason every man over the age of forty should have an annual (and after age fifty, semiannual) rectal examination of the prostate by his personal physician. Other screening tests are currently being evaluated, but most cancer experts agree that the simple digital rectal examination remains essential.

2

THE UROLOGICAL
EXAMINATION

Years ago, family doctors would sometimes say, "Oh, aside from his urological problem, he's in good shape." But that assessment is too vague, because sometimes a patient may look well but have many physical problems. Former mayor Jimmy Walker of New York City used to say: "You can walk by a building, and the outside may be well painted and beautiful, but the plumbing inside can be in lousy shape." That holds true for people, especially when urological problems are involved. A man may have a full head of hair, excellent posture, and the appearance of a healthy athlete, yet be running to the bathroom every hour due to prostate trouble.

Fear that surgery may be necessary, as well as a general fear of the unknown, discourages too many men from consulting a urologist when they should. Often, a prostate problem can be handled so simply and speedily that the patient is relieved of his discomfort before he leaves the urologist's office. Still, it is not uncommon for a patient to admit that he has been suffering from symptoms of prostate trouble for months—even years—before finally making the appointment when the pain became unbearable. But why bear such discomfort at all? A urologist can usually help.

Sometimes a man puts off discussing the problem with

any physician until an emergency strikes. Unable to urinate, he has developed what is called *acute retention.* All too often, this happens in the middle of the night. A man may be uncomfortable all evening, having to go to the bathroom constantly and passing just a few drops of urine each time. He does not call a doctor because he fails to realize that he is going to be in real trouble soon. Because passing a few drops of urine offers some relief, the man thinks he is all right; but later, when he is unable to release even those few drops, he finds himself in real agony.

In the days when doctors made home visits, the man's personal physician might have come over to his home and inserted a catheter—a thin, smooth, flexible rubber or plastic tube that can be inserted into the penis, through the urethra, and into the bladder, to drain the urine. Today, a man usually must go to his doctor or (if it is the middle of the night) to the emergency room of his local hospital, where he will be catheterized. Sometimes a patient who hasn't urinated for twelve or fourteen hours may have as much as four quarts of urine removed through the catheter. The emergency room staff or his own doctor will probably suggest that he promptly make an appointment with a urologist to get to the cause of the problem and to prevent future recurrences of this unpleasant experience.

Urinary retention usually occurs because of some sort of prostate obstruction, although other conditions (as well as certain drugs) can cause it, too. Men in their sixties or seventies should not take antihistamines or decongestants on a regular basis, because they can cause a contraction of the smooth muscle that surrounds the bladder neck and prostate, as well as relaxing the bladder muscle itself, resulting in a urinary shutdown. Antihistamines usually do not have this effect in younger people, but anyone who experiences narrowing of the bladder neck and prostate problems may find antihistamines problematic. Too much alcohol, particularly beer, also can cause acute retention.

Most men who come to the urologist's office are not experiencing an acute episode but have been sent by their personal physician for a more complete diagnosis and for possible treatment. The following outline of a typical urological examination offers a realistic (and reassuring) description of the simplicity and relative painlessness of the experience.

COMPILING A COMPLETE HISTORY

The first thing a urologist will do is compile a complete medical and social history. The patient is asked general questions about any illnesses or surgery he has had—including illnesses such as mumps, rheumatic fever, and nephritis (kidney disease)—and many specific questions—such as whether he has experienced any swelling in his testicles, and whether his testicles or penis has even been injured.

The patient may be asked about his social habits—how much coffee and liquor he drinks, and what his sexual practices (past and present) are. Naturally, the patient is also given the opportunity to tell the urologist in his own words why he has come to see him, and the urologist makes a complete list of the patient's complaints and symptoms. As a rule, a man comes to see a urologist because he feels pain in the area of his kidneys, back, or genitals, or because of some malfunction, discomfort, or pain he experiences during urination or sexual activity. Of course, in a particular case these symptoms may not be related to any urological condition, but it is up to the urologist to determine if this is so.

If there is a history of diabetes in the patient's family, he should be sure to tell the urologist—if the urologist does not bring up the subject himself. A predisposition to this disease often is inherited and may not surface until later in life. Diabetes can lead to frequent urination, and it can interfere with sexual functioning. It is not unusual for a man to think he has prostate problems when instead, he is manifesting signs of diabetes.

The patient should also tell the urologist if he has ever had any venereal or nonvenereal infection, because these symptoms can cause a stricture in the urethra and result in symptoms similar to those seen in prostate disorders. A venereal disease that has not been completely cured can cause infections in the prostate.

The urologist usually wants to know how often the patient urinates and whether any change has occurred in his usual urinating pattern. By watching the patient urinate, the urologist can observe which of four types of urine stream he produces. It may be a full, normal-size stream. It may be a thin stream that shows a narrowing that could be due to a stricture (narrowing of the urethra) or a prostatic obstruction. It may be a dribble, or the patient may have to "push," suggesting that the obstruction is somewhere in the area of the prostate. Finally, it may be a split stream, in which the stream seems to spray; this symptom is often due to a stricture of the external opening of the tip of the penis.

Many men are self-conscious about urinating in front of anyone—even a doctor—so this method does not always give the urologist an accurate idea of his normal stream. In addition, urologists need to know more than can be learned from observing the stream, so they make use of urodynamics (medical studies of urination). One valuable urodynamic test makes use of a mechanical uroflometer. In this test, the patient urinates into a funnel, and the urine flows into compartments or chambers of the uroflometer, each of which has little holes, calibrated in such a way as to allow the urologist to identify the extent of the peak force of the urine flow. A computerized variant of this test gives additional information by means of a taped readout.

Many methods can be used to determine whether a man is able to empty his bladder completely. Making this determination is important because an inability to empty the bladder completely may be due to prostatic obstruction and may in turn lead to other problems such as infections or kidney disease.

URINALYSIS AND BLOOD TESTS

Prior to examination, a patient is usually asked to leave a sample of urine (often directly into the uroflometer, so the force of the stream can be determined, as well), and in many instances a sample of blood will be drawn from the patient's arm.

A urinalysis, which is performed by dropping special tablets or dipping tapes or small sticks that resemble blotting paper into a urine sample and observing the results, as well as by examining urine under a microscope, reveals much about a person's health. Among the potential abnormalities a urologist looks for in the urine sample are red blood cells, excessive white blood cells, sugar, albumin, and blood cell casts. The presence of red blood cells suggests problems in the urinary tract such as stones or tumors, but it may also result from simple BPH. A large number of white blood cells may indicate an infection of the prostate. The presence of white blood cells or pus may also indicate infection or inflammation in the kidneys, ureters, or bladder. At one time, tuberculosis of the prostate was common. It would begin in the lung or in the bones, and then travel to the prostate. Today, drugs cure TB, so prostatic tuberculosis is rare; but it is still possible, so urologists are careful to check for it. Sugar in the urine may be a sign of diabetes. Albumin (protein substance) and blood cell casts (fibrous material) often indicate kidney problems. The specific gravity of the urine is checked to determine the number of solid particles it contains; the greater the concentration of solid particles, the more proficient the kidneys are at absorbing water and secreting particles. In addition to the immediate urinalysis, a urine culture is sometimes taken to help determine whether infections are present.

A complete blood count (CBC) may be done in the urologist's office, unless the patient's personal physician has just performed one. The CBC will reveal departures from the normal standards (which may indicate general disease) and medical problems that may or may not be related to the urinary tract. Some doctors send their patients to a local commercial laboratory for these tests. A blood urea nitrogen (BUN) test and a serum creatinine level test are performed to measure kidney function. Many urologists routinely do an acid phosphatase test and a serum prostate-specific antigen test on a blood sample because these can give important information about the possibility of cancer.

EXTERNAL PHYSICAL EXAMINATION

The next step is a thorough physical examination, which usually begins with having the patient lie flat on his back. This way the urologist can palpate (examination by feeling with hands) the lower abdomen (to see if the bladder is full), the kidneys, and the abdominal wall. Then the patient sits up, so the doctor can check his back and flanks over each kidney (just under the rib cage), looking for areas of tenderness and for any signs of enlargement.

A man's external genitals are examined most easily when he is standing. The penis and the testes are examined for any structural abnormalities or any signs of infection. The urologist looks for possible cysts, growths, or tumors in the testicles and penis. He carefully checks for a varicocele, an enlargement of veins that can produce what looks like a boggy (that is, soft, spongy, and swollen) tumor of the scrotum; varicocele has been implicated as a cause of infertility. If this arises in later life (fifth or sixth decade), it may be indicative of blockage of the renal vein.

Finally, the urologist checks the overall appearance of the patient, since a severe urological obstruction may manifest itself through weight loss, swelling of the hands and face, a pallor suggestive of anemia, tenderness in kidney areas, a mass in the lower abdomen, or cardiac or pulmonary abnormalities.

DIGITAL RECTAL EXAMINATION

The urologist performs a rectal examination to identify any abnormalities in the anal sphincter or the bladder and to check the prostate itself. The patient bends at the waist and leans over the examination table or chair, while the doctor inserts a well-lubricated, gloved index finger into the rectum. This digital examination is the one part of the examination many men dread, but it is neither painful nor very uncomfortable. Once a man experiences such an examination, he is unlikely to be so anxious the next time.

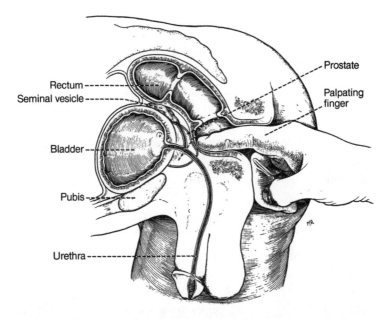

Prostate

Rectum

Seminal vesicle

Palpating finger

Bladder

Pubis

Urethra

The normal prostate feels smooth, elastic, and about the size of a chestnut. When affected by BPH (benign prostatic hypertrophy), the prostate feels similar but larger. Sometimes BPH cannot be diagnosed by examination alone, because the growth occurs into the base of the bladder, but such growth will show up in x-rays or scans.

The urologist, with his trained index finger, can detect various disorders. Most important, he can detect early signs of cancer. He looks for a small, hard nodule or for areas of undue firmness. Chronic infections or stones can mimic the signs of malignancy, but an x-ray or sonogram will often distinguish stones from tumors.

If a urologist suspects cancer, he may perform a number of tests, including (perhaps) a biopsy. This is a minor surgical procedure in which a part of the hard nodule or other tissue is removed, either by needle biopsy or by aspiration, and then subjected to laboratory tests. No matter how convinced a urologist is, based on examination, that a hard nodule is or is not cancer, he cannot be 100 percent certain without laboratory proof. The tests for prostate cancer are discussed in chapter 7.

If physical examination does not reveal any problems and the patient's symptoms are minor, the urologist may order further tests or may simply reassure the patient that he is fine but should have periodic follow-up examinations.

X-RAY EXAMINATION

X-rays remain an important diagnostic tool for urologists, and many do these studies in their own offices. Others send patients to the office of a radiologist for x-rays. If the urologist plans to do it in his own office, patients are often told not to eat or drink anything during the twelve hours prior to a urological appointment. This is because the urologist may take an x-ray that requires him to inject dye into a vein; the dye goes through the bloodstream and is excreted by the kidney. When normal fluid intake is withheld, the urine becomes more concentrated, enabling the dye to reveal more clearly the structure of the kidney, ureter, and bladder. If you will be sent elsewhere for the test, you may be given those same instructions prior to that appointment.

The condition of kidneys and bladder may be revealed in a simple x-ray. If any stones have developed, these will be visible (except for uric acid stones, which do *not* show up clearly in simple x-rays, but do show up in sonograms and IVPs). An x-ray may be taken after the patient has urinated, in which case the picture may show if there is a large residue of urine left in the bladder. If this occurs, it may be because an obstruction (such as an enlarged prostate) is preventing the complete emptying of the bladder.

The urologist sometimes decides to obtain a series of pictures that may be called either an intravenous pyelogram (IVP) or an intravenous urogram (IVU). For this purpose, dye is injected intravenously (through the veins) and passes through the patient's body, outlining the bladder, the ureters, and the kidneys. When the dye gets to the bladder, it reveals enlargement of the prostate (if such exists) by showing the effects of the prostate obstruction on the bladder contour.

The first x-ray film is taken within a minute or so after the dye is injected. Then, depending on what he sees, the urologist or radiologist decides how many more pictures to take and at what intervals. Generally, four more pictures are taken—ten, fifteen, twenty, and thirty minutes after the dye is injected. If the prostate is greatly enlarged, the dye will be delayed in passing through and will probably not show up in the early pictures. Obstructions of various other kinds have a similar effect.

Most people show no reaction to the dye used in an IVP. Others react to it mildly, but some people are strongly allergic to it. If a man has any allergies or asthma, most urologists will avoid doing an IVP in the office or even at a local radiologist's office. Either they use an alternate test or do it in the out-patient department of the hospital where it can be done with greater safety. All precautions are taken to avoid causing allergic reactions, including use of a new dye that affords greater safety for patients who have allergies. In some instances, physicians may administer antiallergy medication or even cortisone prior to the test.

At one time, IVPs were routinely scheduled for all men with prostate complaints or symptoms, but many urologists today prefer to get much of the information they need from ultrasound tests, especially if the patient reports having had problems in the past with allergies.

ULTRASOUND EXAMINATION

Ultrasound (sometimes called ultrasonography or sonography) uses high-frequency sound waves to examine parts of the body. A sonogram or scan is the record of the test. During the test, a wandlike instrument called a transducer is passed back and forth over the area to be examined. The transducer transmits sound waves and receives echoes, which are electronically processed to form a fairly detailed picture on the screen. Once collected, these images can be recorded on paper or x-ray film for future reference. In an examination of the bladder and prostate, the wand is passed over the abdomen while the bladder is distended with urine. The doctor then repeats the test after the man has urinated, to determine if any urine remains in the bladder after it has been "emptied." Ultrasound equipment is available in most hospitals, in radiologist's offices, and in the offices of a growing number of urologists who prefer to conduct the test themselves.

Since ultrasound does not use radiation and does not require the injection of dye or any other material, it is completely painless and harmless; as a result, it can be repeated many times, so that the urologist can measure any prostatic growth or change. For diagnosing problems of the prostate, ultrasound is excellent, and many urologists use it extensively. Some parts of the urinary system, however, are better viewed with an IVP.

A transrectal probe can be used in place of or in addition to the abdominal sonogram just described.

Many urologists and radiologists (physicians who specialize in various kinds of body imaging, including x-rays and sonograms) recommend using transrectal sonograms. A probe, covered with a rubber balloon that is filled with water, is inserted into the rectum to create an ultrasonic image that can be videotaped. Proponents of this test feel that it provides an excellent adjunct to digital examination for detecting prostate cancer. Some experts believe that it can detect small tumors the manual examination misses. Other urologists are less enthusiastic, saying that the test produces many false readings. Still other urologists find the transrectal ultrasound useful for evaluating the size and precise location of a tumor after it has been detected, and as a guide to the biopsy needle (discussed in chapter 7).

MAGNETIC RESONANCE IMAGING (MRI)

Magnetic resonance imaging (MRI) is a noninvasive technique capable of producing a three-dimensional, cross-sectional body image that is even more detailed than the image created by a CAT scan. There is no radiation exposure in this test; instead, radio waves and a magnetic field are used to delineate the tissues. It is still a fairly new and as yet rarely used technique, but it is becoming available in a growing number of communities, and many experts believe that it will someday be very useful in the evaluation of prostatic cancers and their spread.

THE CYSTOSCOPE

The cystoscope is a slim, hollow tube that is inserted into the penis and passes through the urethra into the bladder. At the end of this instrument is a light to illuminate the bladder's interior. By making use of a number of different lenses, the urologist can see the interior of the bladder and can also get a close look at the prostate and urethra. It is even possible to take an x-ray picture or generate a sonogram by this means.

Cystoscopy is seldom necessary in a simple case of prostate enlargement, especially if the rectal examination plus a sonogram or x-ray confirms the diagnosis. If blood is present in the urine, however, and if the scan is not conclusive, a urologist may want to determine by cystoscope if there is a tumor or any other abnormality in the bladder.

Various sizes and designs of cystoscopes can be kept on hand, enabling the urologist to choose the one best suited to each individual patient. Traditionally, the cystoscope was a rigid metal tube but a flexible synthetic one is now widely available, and many urologists make use of this new development. The field of vision is better with the rigid cystoscope, however, so in many instances, it is still used.

Many urologists perform a cystoscopy on patients in order to view the prostate; other urologists only do this under special circumstances, such as to evaluate a patient with hematuria (blood in urine). Even under the most carefully controlled conditions, cystoscopy can introduce an infection. Thus, many urologists never use it only to view the prostate, except in the operating room just prior to surgery.

Cystoscopy has the reputation of being a painful procedure, but it need not be so, even with the rigid cystoscope. That is because urologists today inject a local anesthetic such as Xylocaine into the penis about five to fifteen minutes before they do the cystoscopy, and as a result there is almost no significant pain. All urologists and clinicians use this local anesthetic for men—or should. If anyone wants to perform a cystoscopy on a patient without the anesthetic, the patient has good reason to protest.

Occasionally a patient is so afraid of the cystoscope that he becomes excessively tense and anxious. If a doctor feels that cystoscopy is essential, he will probably either give such a patient a sedative (by mouth or injection) or decide to do the procedure in the hospital under general anesthesia.

The initial visit to a urologist's office usually takes an hour or two. At the conclusion, the doctor should be able to give the patient some idea as to what is causing his problem. Sometimes, depending on the diagnosis, a decision can be made on a beginning course of treatment. If the urologist suspects cancer of the prostate, other diagnostic tests will be scheduled.

If the patient receives a clean bill of urological health from the urologist but his symptoms persist, his personal physician will probably run additional medical tests and refer him to the appropriate specialist to rule out other possible disorders. Regardless of the findings, the urologist will send a written report to the patient's personal physician. Many urologists use what, in the Greenberger office, was always called the "PUP" (Pick Up Phone) system. In the presence of the patient, the urologist speaks to the referring doctor, reporting to him about the tests and examinations that were performed and the findings that resulted. Later the personal physician gets all this in writing, but the immediate communication is helpful to both the patient and his physician. In particular, it reassures the patient that the urologist has been truthful with him and that there are no secrets between the doctors about *his* body. Patients who are handled in this way seem to appreciate it and (perhaps as a result) are very cooperative.

3

INFECTIOUS PROSTATITIS: ACUTE AND CHRONIC

Prostatitis—whether acute or chronic—is an inflammation of the prostate so common that every man, from teenager to golden-ager, should be prepared for the possibility of its occuring at any time. Because prostatitis is so uncomfortable, it may at first seem more serious to the patient than it really is. In fact, however, the condition responds well (although often slowly) to treatment.

Infection, irritation, congestion, or a combination of these problems can cause prostatitis. Sometimes the cause cannot be determined. The treatments vary, depending on the precise diagnosis. This chapter discusses infectious prostatitis, both acute and chronic.

ACUTE CASES VERSUS CHRONIC CASES

Few problems will send a man to his doctor faster than acute prostatitis—and small wonder. It is usually signaled by a sudden onset of fever, chills, nausea, and vomiting, in addition to numerous difficulties associated with urination (urgency, hesitancy, burning, pain, and pus or blood in the urine). If his personal physician suspects acute prostatitis, he will probably send the patient to a urologist for a complete diagnosis.

Chronic prostatitis often follows a case of arrested (but not completely cured) acute prostatitis, although it can exist without ever having been acute. It ranges from a mild, almost symptom-free state to a state of extreme discomfort, often accompanied by a urinary tract infection. Fever seldom accompanies chronic prostatitis. A man with chronic prostatitis feels an uncomfortable fullness in the rectum, rather than pain, but the condition is certainly unpleasant enough to cause him eventually to seek help.

Chronic prostatitis is frustrating for both patient and urologist because, often when the patient has just begun to feel better, the symptoms start up again. Even the most loyal patient begins to wonder if he should see another urologist, and many patients do. Any well trained, ethical urologist they consult will explain, however, that in many cases chronic prostatitis is never really cured, and that the best any doctor can hope to do is to keep the patient comfortable and relatively symptom-free in remission for extended periods of time.

Men with chronic prostatitis commonly worry that they are more likely to develop BPH or cancer of the prostate than other men. On the contrary, they may have a better chance of avoiding *serious* trouble from these diseases, since they see a urologist regularly who is quick to recognize the earliest stage of BPH or cancer *if* it occurs.

CAUSES OF INFECTION

Infectious prostatitis is caused by bacteria or other microorganisms that have found their way into the prostate via the bloodstream, the lymph system, the penis, or the urethra. The most common prostatic infection comes from bacteria that are in the colon. Since the advent of antibiotics, this form of infection poses less of a problem than it once did; if an infection does take hold, it can usually be cured before it becomes too serious. Prostatitis from infection can also be sexually transmitted: *Trichomonas vaginalis, Candida albicans* (yeast infection), and gonorrhea can be transmitted from a woman during sexual activity and result in acute prostatitis. Occasionally, a viral or bacterial infection may not reveal itself in cultures and under the microscope, simply because the tests used are still not sufficiently sophisticated to identify *all* infections.

The prostate resides in a capsule that is not easily penetrated and is fairly well protected against infectious organisms in the system. But when such organisms *do* find their way in, they discover a very hospitable host. Because the prostate does not drain itself well, the infection can easily take hold and may be difficult to evict.

Certain substances in the diet can cause a type of chronic prostatitis in some people. Among the foods under suspicion are coffee, gin, scotch whiskey, and red wine. The flavorings in these drinks contain significant amounts of aromatic oils that can irritate the prostate. Although these beverages are not likely to cause an initial attack of prostatitis, a man who has had prostate problems is susceptible to their effects.

Safer sex is the best insurance against all sexually transmitted infections. Unless you are in a truly monogamous relationship and know your partner's sexual history, use a condom and avoid oral sex.

At one time, gonorrhea was the most common cause of all major infections of the male urogenital tract. Since the advent of antibiotics, gonorrhea can usually be cured quickly, before it has a chance to travel to the prostate. Occasional abscesses do occur in the prostate, how-often caused by gonorrhea, particularly among men who acquired a drug-resistant strain or ignored prompt treatment. These patients exhibit the same general symptoms that are characteristic of acute prostatitis.

PREVENTING INFECTIOUS PROSTATITIS

Is there some way to prevent infectious prostatitis? Sometimes, yes. Good health practices are important in preventing any bacterial infection. Advice not to drink unsafe water should always be heeded. Aside from the miserable stomach upsets that can result, contaminated water can introduce dangerous bacteria to any part of the body, including the prostate.

A man who does develop an infection anywhere in his body should be sure to have it promptly and fully treated. If a doctor tells a patient to take an antibiotic for ten days, he must not stop taking it before the full ten days have passed just because he is feeling better. The prescribed treatment time is the minimum time required to ensure destruction of all the infectious bacteria. Shortening the treatment time only invites a prompt resurgence of the bacteria.

DIAGNOSING AND TREATING INFECTIOUS PROSTATITIS

When a patient suffers from what appears to be acute infectious prostatitis, the urologist is extremely cautious in his examination of the prostate, because too much pressure might spread the infection to the testicles, epididymus, or bloodstream, causing severe systemic infection. To determine the appropriate antibiotic to prescribe, the prostate is palpated gently (if at all), in order to release some of the prostatic fluid for microscopic examination. (This fluid is expelled through the urethra and penis.) Many urologists *never* perform a rectal examination on a man with these symptoms; *no* urologist ever presses the prostate vigorously under these circumstances.

When the infection is acute (and often the first time the symptoms are noticed, it is acute), it usually clears up dramatically in response to antibiotics and other supportive treatments: liquids, pain relievers, stool softeners, and rest. Only in severe cases where the prostate does not respond to the treatment quickly is hospitalization necessary. If a patient is unable to urinate, it may be necessary to remove urine directly from his bladder by means of an aspiration needle or catheter inserted through the lower abdomen—rather than inserted through the urethra, since this could exacerbate the problem. The infection *will* clear up, but a urologist can never say with certainty that he has cured it, since these infections have a tendency to recur as uncomfortable and bothersome chronic conditions.

Men with chronic prostatitis become adept at recognizing symptoms of a flareup at an early stage, and should call their doctor before they become really ill. A man who is alert to his own body is wise. Although people shouldn't try to treat themselves (even doctors should not do this!), an educated patient notices differences in the way his body is behaving and recognizes when something is wrong, even if he does not know what that something is.

Some people, for no known reason, seem to have a susceptibility to developing chronic prostatitis. Doctors always hope that the latest antibiotic will offer a lasting cure for this persistent problem. But too often the bacteria infecting the prostate become immune to the effects of the drug, or the drug does not concentrate satisfactorily in the prostate. New drugs are regularly introduced, however, and some work very well. Sitz baths offer relief, but there is yet no completely satisfactory drug treatment for chronic prostatitis.

Some urologists believe that one effective treatment for chronic prostatitis is for the doctor to massage the prostate at regular intervals. Other urologists are far less enthusiastic about this procedure, and some do not believe in it at all. To perform such a massage, the physician simply inserts a gloved finger into the rectum and strokes the prostate very gently. The physiological effect of prostatic massage is essentially the same as that of sexual intercourse or masturbation: to relieve the symptoms of chronic prostatitis by draining accumulated prostatic fluid from the glands and ducts.

Urologists generally feel that regular sexual activity of any type leading to ejaculation is the best way to empty the prostate of fluid, but for one reason or another this is not an alternative available or acceptable to everyone. As many more men remain single and grow increasingly concerned about the implications of safer sex, prostatic massage may have a resurgence in urological offices. Certainly, sexual activity is an excellent urological (as well as general physical and psychological) prescription for all human beings, but the Greenberger office associates never believed it was the *only* prescription for a prostate that needs to be drained.

A woman with a sexually transmittable infection should tell her partner about it because (particularly with *Trichomonas vaginalis,* which may go unnoticed in the male) he, too, should be treated. Otherwise, these ailments tend to be passed back and forth between partners. Any change a man notices on his penis—skin eruptions, for example—should be brought to the attention of his physician at once. Treating the problem at its inception may prevent it from causing prostatitis. Some sexually transmitted conditions can be treated locally with an antibiotic cream or ointment; others require oral medication.

Before modern drugs and antibiotics were developed, prostate abscesses were more common and were difficult to treat; they usually had to be incised. Today, if antibiotics are not successful in clearing up an abscess in the prostate, the doctor may surgically incise it, entering through the penis and urethra or (in some cases) through the rectum. This is a relatively minor procedure, but it must be done under anesthesia.

A favorite story in the Greenberger family involves Mary-Ellen, who at the age of nine was already practicing to be a social worker. One evening as her parents were returning from dinner, they heard her on the phone saying: "Oh, Mrs. Jones, I know your husband is in pain and I'm sorry, but my dad's out for dinner. Now if you will just run a nice hot bath for your husband and tell him to sit in it, he will feel much better, and by that time my dad will be home. He would only tell you the same thing and then remind you to bring your husband into the office first thing in the morning. But if you don't trust *me,* call back later."

Sitz baths are as old as urology and are a home remedy that urologists still recommend. A sitz bath (really just an ordinary hot tub bath) uses the heat from the water to increase circulation to the affected area. Sitz baths have long been a good first-aid treatment for many urinary retention problems, and they are also used as one aspect of treatment for acute prostatitis, chronic prostatitis, and BPH. Most urologists suggest sitz baths if a patient is having trouble urinating, but if he is experiencing severe pain or acute retention (pain from an inability to urinate at all), he should see a doctor as soon as possible.

SURGERY

Some people ask why a urologist does not simply end a case of chronic prostatitis by removing the prostate. One way to answer this question is to compare chronic prostatitis with tonsilitis. Some people get frequent mild attacks of tonsilitis, with an occasional acute attack; yet most doctors do not advise surgery for tonsilitis, unless a person regularly has acute attacks. And even in the latter case, tonsils are never removed during an acute attack; instead, surgery takes place after the present bout of tonsilitis ends.

In the same way, prostatitis seldom is treated surgically. Occasionally, if a case of chronic prostatitis becomes intolerable to the patient, or if it causes urinary retention or kidney problems, surgery may be performed—but not during an acute stage. Afterward, the inflammation and infection may persist in the prostatic capsule, despite removal of the prostate itself.

A man who has frequent infections of the prostate has a tendency to develop stones (precipitated mineral solids) in the gland, which then become contaminated, perpetuating the prostate infection. Likewise, a man with one or more stones in his prostate has a tendency to develop infections. Since medical treatment alone seldom removes the contamination from the stones, surgery may be necessary in this instance. The surgery is usually a fairly simple form of closed surgery called *transurethral resection* (TUR). This procedure is described in detail in chapter 6.

Many people wonder if the stones can be crushed by a

lithotriptor—a recently developed machine that crushes stones in the kidney and ureter, allowing them to be passed through the urethra and avoiding surgery. Unfortunately, because the prostate is enclosed in a capsule, these stones would not have any route out of the body if they were crushed. Consequently, this excellent new method does not, at its present stage of technological development, work for stones in the prostate.

Although prostate infections (whether acute or chronic) are uncomfortable, they *are* treatable, and effective new medications are constantly being developed. A man who suffers from prostatitis does need to be patient, but in time he will feel better.

NONINFECTIOUS PROSTATITIS

When a patient complains of lower-back pain, pelvic discomfort, a burning feeling in his penis during urination, urinary urgency or frequency, discomfort or pain after ejaculation, or hematospermia (slight bleeding with ejaculation), it is likely that his problems are related to the prostate. If a doctor has ruled out bacterial infection as the cause and has noted (during a rectal examination) that the prostate is soft, boggy, and filled with prostatic fluid but does not seem to be enlarged or to have any hard nodules, he will suspect that the patient is suffering from noninfectious prostatitis and will refer him to a urologist.

CONGESTIVE PROSTATITIS AND PROSTATODYNIA (IRRITATIVE PROSTATITIS)

Urologists do not agree about why some men suffer from a form of noninfectious prostatitis characterized by congestion of the prostate and an inflammatory condition. Studies inquiring into its cause have been inconclusive, although it is believed to result either from an infectious disease caused by an as yet unidentified organism or from some noninfectious form of inflammation.

Veteran urologists have noted that, when a patient suffering from this type of prostatitis is examined rectally, a great deal of prostatic fluid is expelled through the urethra and penis, and many patients express relief almost immediately. Why is this?

Each day the normal prostate of a healthy man secretes about $\frac{1}{10}$ to $\frac{2}{5}$ teaspoon of prostatic fluid. This small amount is readily passed off with the man's urine. When a man is sexually aroused, however, production of prostatic fluid increases to four to ten times that amount, providing a component of seminal fluid to help carry the sperm cells through the urethra and expel them at the man's sexual climax. When arousal is not followed by ejaculation, the fluid manufactured to meet the anticipated demand remains in the prostate—although some of this fluid may be expelled if a man has frequent nocturnal emissions. If prostatic fluid continues to accumulate in the prostate, it is easy to understand how the congestion it causes in the prostate can bring a man to a point of discomfort and lead to one or more of the symptoms described at the beginning of this chapter.

Many men who suffer from congestive prostatitis find that their sexual habits (or lack of them) are at the root of the problem. In cases where this is not so, the urologist must consider other possible explanations. For example, some men seem to produce more than the usual amount of prostatic fluid and fail to ejaculate all of it at climax. For such a man, treatment may have to proceed on a trial-and-error basis, but generally he can be afforded some relief.

Some men suffer the symptoms of prostatic congestion—particularly a sense of pelvic heaviness or pain—but the examination shows no signs of congestion, and other studies reveal no urological problems. These men may suffer from prostatodynia, once referred to as irritative prostatitis. Patients with prostatodynia have symptoms that seem to be the same as either infectious or noninfectious (congestive) prostatitis; the predominant symptom is pelvic pain. It is mainly seen in men twenty to forty-five years old. Some patients have urinary urgency, frequency, and some of the signs of an obstructive problem, such as hesitancy and a weakened urinary stream.

Upon examination, however, these men show no signs of any abnormality. There is no history of infections of the prostate and no evidence that the prostate is congested.

At this time, no definitive cause of this condition has been established. Some urologists believe that the perineal muscles may be fatigued, others believe that stress is clearly implicated, and some feel that irritation is the cause. The Greenberger files are full of stories about men whose prostate problems are difficult to explain—without a full understanding of their life-style.

Treating a patient who has noninfectious prostatitis is difficult because the underlying cause is not definitively established. Antibiotics are often helpful, however, and are frequently prescribed for short periods of time. Normal sexual activity and exercise are encouraged, and hot sitz baths provide effective relief of symptoms. Men who have discomfort when urinating often feel better if they take certain medications that are designed to work directly on muscles of the bladder, or if they take antiinflammatory drugs such as ibuprofen. Although oral zinc is often suggested for this purpose, its effectiveness has not been proved.

When a patient fails to make a speedy recovery (and often patients do not recover quickly), he may become a "doctor shopper," looking for a surgeon who is willing to do exploratory surgery in search of some undiscovered abnormality that might be causing the symptoms. Such surgery is unlikely to reveal anything.

When confronted with a case where a man shows symptoms of prostatic congestion but no physical evidence of it, a urologist may look for an underlying psychological cause. Great anxiety or stress-related tensions about job, family, or school (not just about sex) can produce these symptoms. Sometimes if the man discusses some of these stresses with the urologist, reassurance that his symptoms will cease is enough to give relief. If the patient's symptoms are not relieved, the urologist may refer him to a psychiatrist, psychologist, social worker, or minister for counseling or to learn stress-reduction techniques. But it is bad policy to rush a patient off for emotional counseling until all bodily symptoms have been fully investigated by the physician.

Sometimes a condition responds best to a combination of physical *and* emotional treatment. For this reason, urologists often work closely with people from other helping professions and refer patients to many of them. Conversely, a social worker or psychologist might refer someone to a urologist because the patient has revealed problems with sexuality that raise the possibility of a urological problem.

For example, a man might complain to his psychologist that often, when he is talking to a pretty woman at a cocktail party, he has to excuse himself to go to the bathroom and urinate. He may simply be manifesting anxiety about talking to a woman. But the wise psychologist knows that the patient may in fact be suffering from prostate problems. Only when his frequent need to urinate interferes with pleasurable experiences does he become aware that he seems to have a urological problem. A urologist can clarify the matter. Such a case emphasizes why urologists need to obtain a full medical, social, and sexual history of each patient and why patients should be as honest and detailed as possible in giving their history.

CASE HISTORIES

Following are descriptions of some patients, their sexual habits, and the treatments suggested for the forms of noninfectious prostatitis that led to their complaints. Cumulatively, these examples demonstrate the importance of giving the urologist a detailed account of the patient's habits and circumstances. Although these case histories are culled from the Greenberger files, all identifying factors have been changed to preserve the individuals' privacy.

Temporary Abstention

Herbert was a fifty-year-old attorney in good general health who enjoyed a twice-weekly game of squash at his local club. He drank moderately and watched his weight carefully. Marjorie, his wife of twenty-five years was recovering from a hysterectomy that followed months of serious gynecological problems. Until the onset of her illness, they had had an active sexual relationship. As Herbert put it rather wistfully, "I always was pleased to know I spent more time making love to Marjorie in a week than I did playing squash, but it's certainly not that way anymore." In the months prior to Marjorie's surgery, they had had sexual relations only occasionally; and at the time he sought a urological consultation, she was still not feeling well enough for sex.

Herbert was suffering from some of the same symptoms as his older brother, who had recently had surgery for BPH. He assumed that he was developing the same condition, but upon examination he was assured that this was not the case at all; to the contrary, his prostate was soft, boggy, and clearly congested. Because there was no infection, his prostate was massaged on his first office visit, and he was pleasantly surprised to find that he felt almost immediate relief.

Why did this help? wondered Herbert. The explanation offered was that a prostate becomes "programmed" for a certain sexual pace. When Herbert abruptly changed his pace, his prostate was unprepared for the change and continued to produce far more fluid than he could use. The result was painful congestion. According to many urological textbooks, the efficacy of prostatic massage has no scientific basis, but there are a number of similar cases in the Greenberger files (as well as in the files of other practicing urologists) to support the belief that it works.

As a devoted husband, Herbert could pursue any of several courses in dealing with his congested prostate: he could ask his wife to help him ejaculate by manual or oral means, he could masturbate, or he could continue to see the urologist or his personal physician for prostatic massage. It was clear that Herbert absolutely would not consider seeking any other sex partner; and such a suggestion from a physician would in any case have been highly inappropriate. Regular ejaculation obviously would be helpful (since one massage had drained his now congested prostate), but the means to achieve this were left up to Herb.

Unrelieved Excitation

Robert, a good-looking high school senior called the urologist's office early Monday morning, complaining of severe pain in the pelvic area, which he had first noticed on Sunday morning (the day before). The urological examination revealed no problems, except a rather congested prostate. Experienced urologists have seen many Roberts in their offices—and often on Monday mornings. Their stories are strikingly similar.

This young man had been going steady with a lovely young woman whose ambitions were similar to his: to go to a good college and someday enter government or law. They usually spent Saturday evenings at her house; if she happened to be babysitting, he would join her on the job. They talked, watched some television, and then found their way to a comfortable couch.

Naturally they would get sexually excited, and Robert (like most young men) would quickly arrive at the brink of orgasm. This couple's moral standards and value system, however, prevented Robert's arousal from being relieved by permitting him an ejaculation or his girlfriend an orgasm. Later, at home, Robert would take a cold shower and go to sleep. (A warm bath would probably have been better; it might have relieved him of some of the congestion in his prostate.) The next morning, Robert would wake up with painful and swollen testicles.

Robert went to the urologist for help and answers, like hundreds of Roberts before him. The prescription: warm baths. The real difficulty, though, related to advising him on how to prevent this problem from arising the next Sunday and the Sunday after that. No responsible physician would suggest that Robert and his girlfriend widen their relationship to provide him with an ejaculatory experience. Logically, the urologist could advise him to relieve his discomfort by masturbating before going to sleep on Saturday night, but even this might not fit into Robert's personal code of behavior.

In this situation, a sensitive urologist explores the

patient's feelings, in addition to explaining what caused the problem. Often the patient himself will suggest an appropriate "prescription," and sometimes the patient needs time to think over his options. It is important that he understand the cause of the problem, be aware of alternative treatment plans, and decide on one that makes him comfortable. Some people do not need direction; they simply need medical permission to do what they wish to do. An experienced urologist tries to relate to each patient in a way that is flexible, accepting, and nonjudgmental, leaving the door open for continued consultation if it should prove to be necessary.

Change of Pace

Another Monday morning call came from Bob. Tall, blond, and handsome, Bob was captain of the tennis team, a member of the school chorus, and popular with all his classmates. He was a smiling, confident young fellow who would make any parent proud. After a moment or two in the office, he confessed that he was scared. He was suffering from pelvic pain, trouble with urination, urgency, and a weakened stream. He was sure he had picked up a venereal disease and wanted to be checked out. All the tests were negative. The diagnosis: prostatodynia.

It was not difficult to identify the cause of the trouble. Bob had been dating Cheryl, a girl who played on the tennis team with him, and they had spent the weekend before the consultation together. (Her parents had had to go out of town, but she had stayed home to play a tennis match.) Bob reported that he had climaxed three times on Friday night, three times on Saturday morning, and then four times on Sunday.

The urologist informed Bob that the prostate cannot

suddenly be expected to work overtime efficiently, after being virtually idle or working only a half-time schedule. Bob was asked what would happen if he were to play five sets of tennis after a long layoff from the sport. He responded that he would not be surprised if his muscles became stiff and uncomfortable and his hand developed blisters from gripping the racquet. It was easy for him to see why his prostate, unprepared to produce the amount of fluid for several ejaculations, was signaling its fatigue and discomfort. His prostate, unlike those of the men discussed previously, was *not* congested. But it certainly was irritated.

It was not necessary to suggest to Bob that he limit his sexual activity (or at least to pace himself more evenly): he came to that conclusion on his own. In the meantime, Bob was told to rest and take warm baths, and aspirin. Before Bob left, he agreed to have a talk with Cheryl. If this much sexual activity were unusual for her, she might be suffering from another common genital disorder, a bladder infection called "honeymoon cystitis." If so, she would be well advised to seek treatment from a urologist or gynecologist.

Young women are highly susceptible to these bladder infections because their vaginal opening is often small and because the penile thrusting during intercourse (particularly with the man on top) occurs along the roof of the vagina—which is actually the first floor of the urethra and bladder. Bacteria present in the vagina are easily pushed into the urethra and bladder by this prolonged activity. Within a few days, the suddenly sexually active woman may be acutely miserable with a bladder infection marked by frequent, burning urination and (occasionally) some blood in the urine.

Feast or Famine

Alan was a captain in the Merchant Marines. He came into the office with the all-too-familiar symptoms of prostatitis. He was a ruddy-faced, thirty-five-year-old married man in good health, with no evidence of bacterial or structural abnormalities in his genitourinary system. But he said his symptoms had persisted, on and off, for the last year. The pain in his rectal area was becoming more intense, and that was why he had made the appointment. He suspected cancer because he had seen some television commercials warning about it and recommending that all men have rectal examinations. Alan was quickly assured that there was no evidence of any malignancy, but that his prostate was soft, boggy, and probably congested. Alan's occupation gave a clue to his problem. His sexual activity was "feast or famine," and this habit was playing havoc with his prostate's programming.

When he was at home (in a midwestern city), Alan and his wife had an intense period of sexual activity. They had a fine relationship; he was not the "girl in every port" type of seaman and had no further sexual activity until he returned home. The feast on shore and the famine at sea, however, were too much for his prostate. It would continue to produce more fluid than Alan could use at sea, so the fluid would accumulate and the prostate would become congested.

Alan's congestion was relieved at the urologist's office in New York City, but that would not be of much help to him while he was on duty. Alan might have looked for some other sexual outlet—extramarital sex or masturbation—but after bringing up these alternatives himself, he said he was not interested in either option. So he was

43

given a list of reputable urologists in each of his regular ports of call so that he could see them and discuss the possibility of prostatic massage.

Although most urologists consider prostatic massage a poor substitute for intercourse as a means of emptying the prostate, the procedure does empty the prostate when it has become painfully congested. It may well be the *only* way to empty it thoroughly so that the man can enjoy sexual relations. Once the symptoms have been eliminated, regular sexual activity (ending in ejaculation) is just the thing to keep the urologist away, at least where congested prostatitis is concerned.

Chronic Vibration

Nothing in John's sexual history indicated a reason for the clear case of congestive prostatitis he exhibited upon examination. Forty-two years old, he was married to a woman of the same age, and they had a regular, fulfilling sexual relationship. The likely cause of John's problem came to light when he said he was a bus driver. Urologists have long noted that men whose occupations expose them to chronic vibration are prone to developing congestive prostatitis. Although the vibration may not be experienced by the patient as sexually stimulating, it is perceived by the prostate that way! In response, the prostate secretes fluid, in keeping with its normal function. Because this fluid is not always expelled as quickly as it accumulates (even if the man is sexually active), the prostate tends to become congested. Men who work as truck drivers, motorcycle policemen, tractor drivers, and railroad workers fall into this group of people whose jobs predispose them to congestive prostatitis. The treatment: more frequent emptying of the prostate, by whatever means is acceptable to John.

Coitus Interruptus

When Frank came to the office, he had all the symptoms of prostatitis, but lab tests failed to show any bacteria. Frank's social and medical history suggested the cause. He came from a large, religious family, and he and his wife (both age thirty-five) already had five youngsters. Five were enough, Frank said, but he and his wife were reluctant to use any type of contraceptive device. So after their fifth child (now in kindergarten) was born, they began relying on coitus interruptus—the interruption of sexual intercourse by withdrawing the penis from the vagina before ejaculation—to limit the size of their family.

Coitus interruptus is the most widely used method of birth control in the world, because it requires no advance planning, medical supervision, or expense. It is also one of the most unreliable methods, because prior to ejaculation a man often dribbles some semen containing enough sperm to impregnate a fertile woman. Coitus interruptus can cause prostatitis, because it disrupts the normal body rhythm and may even diminish the volume of ejaculation.

When this was explained to Frank and his wife, Catherine, who joined him in the consultation room, Frank was troubled. He admitted that he had not been happy with this form of birth control, but he was in a quandary about what else to do. The couple accepted the suggestion that they speak with Catherine's gynecologist about a modified rhythm plan. They felt that since they liked frequent and regular sex, they might be able to rely on the coitus interruptus method only on those days when she believed she was fertile. Frank came to the office from time to time after that, and the method appeared to be working for them. No more pregnancies, no severe prostatic problems, *and* he and his wife were happy. These days, relatively few people in the United States practice coitus interruptus for contraception, but a urologist occasionally sees a man whose wife wishes him to withdraw before ejaculation. Such couples may benefit from a referral to counseling, because they often have other problems, both in and out of the marriage bed.

Coitus Prolongus

Jim and his wife, Jane, were on slightly different sexual timetables, as many couples are. Jim was ready to climax about ten minutes after he began sexual intercourse, while Jane needed more time to reach orgasm. Both Jim and Jane took great pleasure in her pleasure, as well as his, so they worked out a system according to which Jim would hold back when he felt ready to ejaculate, in order to be able to continue thrusting until his wife reached orgasm. This had been their pattern for many years, and it was satisfying for them. But this practice of coitus prolongus, as it is called, led to irritation of Jim's prostate, and it finally sent him to a urologist. The prescription: take warm sitz baths, and allow ejaculation to occur spontaneously. But adopting that suggestion on its own would have left Jane unsatisfied. She might eventually have ended up in a doctor's office complaining of pelvic congestion caused by constant stimulation that did not culminate in orgasm.

Here was a couple with no emotional problems. What they needed was sexual education, rather than marital or sexual therapy. Because they were neither experimental nor aware of the various alternatives for achieving sexual satisfaction, Jim and Jane had relied exclusively on sexual intercourse as the means for Jane to reach orgasm. They were very receptive to the suggestion that Jim might stimulate Jane orally and manually. They looked upon the mention of this educational information as permission from an authority. Indeed it was: not a prescription, merely permission.

A few months later Jim reported that their sex life was happier than ever before, proving once again that some people simply need the opportunity to discuss problems with a knowledgeable physician in an unhurried atmosphere.

The preceding cases point out a number of instances in which certain sexual behaviors contribute to the development of noninfectious prostatitis. But it should be remembered that many men who follow the same practices used by the men in the case studies *never* exhibit any signs of prostatitis. It should also be noted that some men develop congestive prostatitis or prostatodynia for no discoverable reason. Anti-inflammatory drugs are often successful in treating these men, as well as in treating men whose lifestyles may be contributing to their problem.

A word of caution to anyone who might decide to live with the symptoms (regardless of their cause) rather than to seek help: Some evidence indicates that noninfectious prostatitis can make a man more susceptible to infectious prostatitis. This, as explained earlier, can lead to chronic prostatitis—a treatable, but often incurable condition. Neither infectious nor noninfectious prostatitis, however, increases a man's chance of developing BPH or cancer of the prostate. They are separate entities, and no studies have shown any relation among them.

5

ENLARGEMENT OF THE PROSTATE: BPH

Even if you have avoided prostate trouble through most of your adult life, you are not safe from it when you reach your retirement years. At this time of life, even the healthiest man is likely to develop a condition called *BPH (benign prostatic hypertrophy)*. BPH is an enlargement of the glandular tissue within the prostate capsule. Although the condition neither spreads nor attacks other tissues or cells in the body (which is why it is called benign, rather than malignant or cancerous), the enlargement of the affected tissues can push the prostate outward and narrow the urethra. As it presses against other structures it can cause problems ranging from the minor discomforts of nocturia (waking up at night to urinate) and urinary frequency to conditions as serious as uremia (an excess of wastes in the blood) and renal failure (nonfunctioning kidney). Most men tend to ignore the first minor discomforts, but few leave their BPH untreated to the point of almost complete kidney shutdown. The location (rather than the size) of the enlargement determines whether a man will experience symptoms.

CAUSES OF BPH

Attempts to identify risk factors in men who eventually develop BPH have not been successful. There is no relationship to celibacy, specific blood groups, use of tobacco or alcohol, coronary heart disease, hypertension, exposure to chronic vibration, or any other condition. Approximately 50 percent of all men develop some enlargement of the prostate by the age of sixty. Among eighty-year-old men, only some 5 percent have not developed symptoms of BPH.

The only men who, as a group, *do* seem to escape this fate are those who have been castrated (had their testicles removed surgically or shrunk through intake of female hormones). For this reason, scientists believe that enlargement of the prostate gland is somehow related to the production and presence of male hormones. While hormones may not *cause* BPH, two major factors are clearly necessary in order for the condition to develop: the presence of the testicles, and aging.

The incidence of BPH in Asian men had long been thought to be very low, but later it was noted that the incidence of both BPH and cancer of the prostate was significantly increased among Asian men who had moved to the West or changed from their traditional life-style. No study has clearly demonstrated why (or even definitely if) this occurs, but it is thought to be related to environment, with diet the most likely cause. Asians traditionally have had a low-cholesterol and low-meat diet; American men might be wise to make a logical connection here and minimize their chances of developing prostate problems (as well as heart disease and other health problems) by limiting the cholesterol and fats in their diet.

One practice that has been implicated in the development of BPH is the use of anabolic steroids by athletes and others who are active in body building. These drugs are sometimes taken in doses many times greater than the maximum amount approved by the Food and Drug

Administration. The abuse of anabolic steroids can also cause breast enlargement in men, atrophied testicles leading to fertility problems, and impotence.

Many patients with BPH ask if anything in their past history could have caused this disorder. The answer is that sexual habits and infections appear to have no effect on the growth of the prostatic glandular tissue. Currently, no clear evidence exists to show how to avoid this growth, although it does appear that the trace mineral zinc is somehow related to the health of the prostate.

SYMPTOMS AND DIAGNOSIS OF BPH

Because the degree of discomfort and pain a person feels is such a subjective matter and because symptoms tend to develop gradually, it is important to bring even the earliest symptoms of BPH to the attention of a doctor.

The usual symptoms of BPH resemble those of other prostatic disorders:

- Hesitancy to begin urination
- Diminution of caliber and force of urinary stream
- Inability to abruptly stop urination; instead, continuing to dribble
- Feeling that the bladder has not been completely emptied
- Urinary frequency, including nocturia (because the bladder is not emptied during previous urination)
- Urinary retention (inability to urinate)
- Nausea, dizziness, or unusual sleepiness (*if* kidneys are damaged)

The diagnosis of BPH is obvious when the examining physician finds the prostate soft, rubbery, and enlarged.

Often an experienced urologist can even estimate the size of the prostate on the basis of this examination.

The effects of BPH vary, and so do the treatments prescribed. In deciding on a course of treatment, the physician considers the general health, age, and life-style of each patient. Years ago men in their sixties or early seventies often expected to experience diminishing health at that age and were not optimistic about relief for their prostate conditions. But in January of 1987, seventy-six-year-old President Ronald Reagan frankly admitted that his prostate was enlarged and underwent surgery, and all over America people saw how quickly he was able to return to his usual routine. Many men in his age group realized, perhaps for the first time, that this common condition need not limit a man's life-style.

CASE HISTORIES

Again (as in chapter 4), case histories from the Greenberger office's files offer representative examples of how BPH is experienced, diagnosed, and treated.

Acute Retention of Urine

Some men, still young in every way, are so involved with their business and family life that they ignore the first symptoms of BPH and eventually suffer such acute retention that they must enter the hospital on an emergency basis to get relief.

Paul was such a patient. The growth of his prostate was so slow that he was unaware of the developing symptoms. He did have to get up a few times each night to urinate, but he expected that to be necessary at sixty-three. He had just expanded his business, and his oldest daughter had recently made him a grandfather for the second time. With all his added responsibilities, he simply did not take time for the usual checkup.

One wintry Saturday night, Paul was in agony, feeling a powerful need to urinate but being unable to do so. Paul was suffering from acute retention. He called his physician, who directed him to the emergency room of the local hospital, where a catheter was inserted into his penis to drain the urine directly from his bladder. It turned out that Paul's bladder had contained over a quart of urine that he had been unable to void. He looked and felt better within minutes after catheterization.

Sudden attacks of acute retention can happen to any man—especially one who has prostatic obstruction. Acute retention often follows exposure to cold, consumption of alcohol, ingestion of cough mixtures that contain antihistamines, or ingestion of antihistamines alone. Doctors working in emergency rooms in college towns often need to treat a few of the "old grads" over the weekend if the school's annual homecoming game falls on a cold November Saturday. Paul's attack was probably precipitated by the long afternoon he spent sitting on a cold park bench while watching his grandson at play. If Paul had had more regular checkups, his growing prostate and its symptoms would have been noted by his personal physician, and he would have been sent to see a urologist long before this acute attack occurred.

Paul's prostate was quite large, weighing almost 60 grams. (A normal prostate weighs 15 to 20 grams.) Often, however, a large prostate does not give a man much discomfort and is not potentially dangerous, because it may not block the passage of urine. On the other hand, sometimes a relatively small prostate (20 grams or so) can cause a great deal of trouble, because it encroaches dangerously upon the urethra, preventing urination.

Although Paul was made comfortable by the removal of the urine in his bladder, he would have had to return to the emergency room soon if the obstacle (the enlargement of the prostate) were not removed. The urologist to whom he was referred ascertained that Paul's general health was good, that he had no infection, and that his prior symptoms were sufficient indication for a prostatectomy. Then he had surgery, and came through it well. In no time he was back at work and enjoying his family, too.

Silent Prostatism

Harry was an elderly married man who had been drowsy, pale, and extremely irritable for several days before suddenly lapsing almost into a coma. He and his wife had mistaken his complaints of tiredness and weakness for normal aspects of aging—which they are not—and had neglected to report his symptoms to Harry's personal physician. Rushed to the hospital in an ambulance, Harry was catheterized in the emergency room; by the next morning, he felt much better.

The problem had been due to benign enlargement of the prostate gland, which had eventually left Harry's bladder full of urine that he could not void. Harry had developed a condition often referred to as *silent prostatism,* in which prostatic obstruction exists but there are no symptoms. The presence of this large amount of unvoidable urine in the bladder had been causing a damaging backflow pressure upon his kidneys, which were near failure when the emergency occurred. A week after the catheter was placed in Harry's bladder, lab results indicated that his renal function had returned to normal. (Some patients' renal function may take up to three months to normalize.) Soon thereafter, Harry's considerably enlarged prostate was surgically removed, and he made a satisfactory recovery.

Because silent prostatism has the potential to do much damage, men over the age of sixty should have annual blood tests that measure kidney function during routine annual physicals.

Enlargement and Congestion

Gerald was in many ways an ideal patient. During his semiannual checkup with his personal physician, he told the doctor that he was concerned because his urinary stream was not as strong as it had been before. Gerald had noticed that, in a public lavatory, the stream no longer reached the back of the urinal. Sometimes, at home, urine would drip on the front rim of the toilet bowl. He was a healthy man who had no other physical problems. His sex life had not changed, but he found this change in urinary pattern sufficiently puzzling to justify reporting it to his doctor. That was a wise step because, even though his doctor routinely performed rectal examinations on all his patients over forty, he was particularly alerted to look for signs of prostatic enlargement when he examined Gerald. The doctor felt some enlargement, but—because it was not very pronounced—he wanted a urologist to evaluate it.

Gerald's urological examination showed some prostatic enlargement, and some mild congestion, but no signs of infection. Tests indicated the existence of some bladder outlet obstruction but also showed that only a small amount of residual urine remained in the bladder after urination. Gerald's kidneys looked fine. Clearly,

Gerald was not in any serious trouble with his prostate at the time of the examination.

If a prostate like Gerald's continues to grow, and the bladder outlet obstruction becomes larger, the bladder will eventually have trouble emptying itself. At some point, the bladder muscle may not be able to keep pace with the obstruction, and it will just give up. The result would be a *decompensated bladder*—one that cannot empty itself. Urine remaining in the bladder causes many of the familiar prostatic symptoms, and it may also leave a man unusually vulnerable to bladder infections. The collecting urine becomes increasingly stagnant and can serve as a perfect culture for growing bacteria. If this happens, the patient will begin to feel burning pain when urinating, and often his urine will have a foul odor. Blood may also appear in the urine if the blood vessels in the bladder stretch so much that they rupture. Depending on the size of the vessel that ruptures, the blood may only slightly color the urine, or it may take the form of a frightening hemorrhage.

The urologist explained all of this to Gerald, saying that he was in no danger of serious trouble at this point, and that sometimes men go through a phase when their prostate bothers them but then causes them no trouble for a long period of time—even without treatment. Studies confirm this observation: many patients who receive no treatment experience no change or exacerbation in symptoms for many years. But Gerald was also told that, because there was evidence of major obstruction at the bladder outlet, he should report any additional symptoms that might arise. He was particularly warned to report immediately if he had any burning upon urination, any chills or fever, or any deterioration in his present symptom, because any of these might indicate a urinary infection. Finally, he was reminded to continue seeing his personal physician regularly, whether he had symptoms or not, and to visit the urologist regularly to ascertain whether any changes had occurred in the interim.

A few weeks later, Gerald reported that, while he was still feeling fairly healthy, he had noticed some additional urinary symptoms, such as nocturia and urgency, and some pelvic heaviness. Upon examination, his prostate felt about the same size as it had before, but it now seemed slightly more congested. As soon as it was massaged and the congested fluid was expelled, the heaviness disappeared. The urologist advised Gerald to consider having regular prostatic massages, which he did. (Other urologists never recommend repeated prostatic massage.)

Gerald's urinary symptoms lessened in response to this treatment, and he was able to avoid surgery for seven years. At that point, Gerald's prostate became much larger, his symptoms increased, and surgery was indicated. He had the simplest surgical procedure (the transurethral resection), and he was able to return to work in a few weeks.

For Gerald and patients like him, many urologists find that prostatic massage is wonderfully therapeutic. For other patients, regular and frequent ejaculation (through intercourse or through masturbation) accomplishes the same results. In addition, men in Gerald's position are wise to avoid prolonged exposure to the cold, to take frequent warm baths, to limit their intake of alcohol and spicy foods, to avoid antihistamines, and to report any increase in symptoms immediately.

WHEN IS SURGERY NEEDED?

Even if the patient's symptoms are mild and there is no kidney impairment, some urologists recommend surgery if a prostate has reached a weight of about 40 grams (twice the normal size). Most urologists, however, prefer to wait until symptoms become severe, or until x-ray studies or sonograms indicate that the patient is not tolerating the enlargement well and is at risk of kidney damage. Occasionally urologists see such massive enlargement of the prostate that it seems remarkable that the patient has managed to void at all. Many cases of BPH fall on a borderline, where surgery might be indicated or the prostate might just be carefully watched.

A urologist considers the individual's life-style in a borderline case. If the patient has no kidney impairment and has a personal reason to want to postpone surgery, he should discuss this with his urologist. The operation can probably wait. President Reagan, for instance, planned his prostate surgery to come at a time that would least interfere with his schedule.

Many men with symptoms of BPH only need reassurance that they do not have cancer and that they are not in imminent danger. In many men, the prostate grows so slowly that it never causes more than minor discomfort. And if the patient does not mind living with the discomfort, why should the patient's doctor object? Still, the patient should continue to be monitored for signs of silent prostatism.

Most patients with BPH report that the condition does not affect their sexual activity, but some, unfortunately, are so concerned that they lose some sexual desire.

It is important to remember that BPH is in *no* way related to cancer of the prostate. BPH is not cancerous and will not turn cancerous; indeed, BPH and cancer of the prostate usually begin in different parts of the prostate. Moreover, a man may have his benign prostatic tissue surgically removed and still develop cancer at some later date. With BPH (unlike with cancer), the growth of the prostate does not do damage in itself; rather, the direction of the growth may cause problems by hindering urination.

Past bouts with bacterial or nonbacterial prostatitis are not a factor in whether or not you develop BPH. Any of these problems can coexist, however, and of course such a compound condition makes both the symptoms and the treatment slightly more complicated.

If the patient is miserable with his symptoms or is at risk of developing kidney impairment, surgery is clearly necessary. Except in some of the urgent situations described previously, though, there is usually no urgency to schedule surgery quickly, so it can be done when most convenient for the patient and his family.

ALTERNATIVE TREATMENTS

The search continues for a treatment other than surgery for benign prostatic hypertrophy. Doctors have known for a long time that castration will prevent (and even cure) BPH, but certainly no doctor would recommend it as a less onerous procedure for this purpose than prostate surgery. Administering female hormones also diminishes the condition, but the side effects of this treatment are most undesirable. Like surgical castration, these female hormones reduce a man's libido (sexual desire), may cause some mild feminization of his body, and often render him impotent. Certainly such a treatment is not preferable to surgery, and it is not common practice except for cancer of the prostate. Occasionally drugs are introduced for the purpose of reducing BPH, but as yet none has proved truly effective for the general population, and some that at first seemed promising have turned out to be disappointing.

Research is currently being conducted on a chemical that blocks an enzyme implicated in the process of prostate enlargement. The studies are an outgrowth of observations that some males born without this specific enzyme never get acne, go bald, *or* develop an enlarged prostate. But commercial availability of this chemical is still a long way off—if indeed work with it ever progresses beyond the testing stage.

At the Mount Sinai School of Medicine in New York City, Michael Droller, M.D., chairman of the Department of Urology, J. Lester Gabrilove, M.D., professor of medicine and a leading endocrinologist, and their colleagues have conducted a study on the effects of a drug called leuprolide on BPH. This drug stimulates production of various hormones that have the same effect on the body as castration. It also shrinks prostate size, and many men who take it experience a significant improvement in urinary symptoms. Shrinkage of the prostate allows urologists to perform a lesser surgical procedure, if one is still needed.

"But," explains Dr. Gabrilove, "any man who takes the drug in doses sufficient to shrink the enlarged prostate will be rendered impotent, and for this reason it is certainly not a drug that would be universally prescribed for BPH. However, this treatment is extremely useful in elderly men whose medical condition is such that they are poor surgical risks and who might already be impotent."

Similar studies indicate that treatments with hormone-blocking drugs—or *antiandrogens,* as they are also known—would have to be maintained indefinitely, since the BPH will redevelop when they are withdrawn. On a more positive note, the impotence would also be reversible.

Although no currently available drug is useful for most men with BPH, researchers hope that future studies will uncover one drug or a combination of drugs that can effectively reduce the enlargement of the prostate without undesirable side effects.

An experimental treatment, now being tested, involves widening the urinary passage by insertion of a balloon. In the procedure, called balloon urethroplasty, a thin, flexible tube is inserted into the penis and guided to the narrowed portion, where the balloon is inflated. The procedure is effective only when the enlargement was from the side lobes of the prostate, and even when it does relieve symptoms it is not yet known when symptoms may reappear.

SURGERY FOR BPH

Surgery! It is hard to face a prostate operation calmly, whether the operation is the patient's first surgical experience or one of many. A prostate operation is different: in the minds of most men, it involves basic masculinity.

The urologist who suggests that the patient have surgery to remove an enlarged prostate usually explains that there is no great rush, but adds that the operation cannot be postponed indefinitely. Over time, the symptoms are likely to worsen.

Some years ago, prostate surgery was a two-stage procedure, and men who underwent it spent weeks on end in the hospital. Since those days, however, prostate surgery has become greatly streamlined.

Three kinds of surgical procedures are most frequently performed to remove prostate glands enlarged as a result of BPH. The surgeon chooses the procedure after considering many factors, particularly the size of the prostate. For smaller prostates, urologists usually choose to perform a transurethral resection of the prostate (TUR or TURP). This procedure is termed a *closed operation* because it is performed without an incision. Instead, a surgical instrument is inserted into the penis and through the urethra, in the same manner as a cystoscope is inserted. The other two procedures, suprapubic prostatectomy and retropubic prostatectomy, are referred to as *open operations.* In these procedures, an incision is made through the skin and fascia below the navel.

Sometimes a urologist may base his choice of procedure on his own preference or area of expertise. A well-trained urologist can perform all three of these procedures with equal skill and will base his choice of method solely on what is best for the patient.

ROUTINE PREPARATIONS FOR SURGERY

Regardless of the surgical procedure planned, some pre-surgical preparations are the same for all patients. In most hospitals, certain routine tests are done, such as an electrocardiogram, a chest x-ray, and blood tests. These routine tests are typically done at the time of admission, often before the patient is assigned to his room. In many hospitals throughout the country, preadmission testing is conducted at some time between a day and a week before admission. The tests specific to the surgery, such as the intravenous pyelogram and sonograms, may have been done prior to the decision for the patient to have surgery. He may be admitted to the hospital on the evening before surgery or, if he is a low-risk patient (a man in good health otherwise), on the day of surgery. Prior to surgery, the urologist will want a medical go-ahead from the patient's personal physician.

After the patient's admission, and before surgery, regular hospital medical staff (the "house staff") often take a medical history of the patient and examine him. This is standard procedure in most hospitals, and the patient's personal physician (and the urologist, too) often relies on these doctors for progress reports between his visits. The patient should feel free to question any procedure of the staff that he has a concern about. At the very least, he can make sure that his doctor has ordered it or is aware of it.

In the patient's room, prior to surgery for any of the open procedures described below, his pubic, scrotal, and abdominal hair is shaved. Some doctors prefer that this be done before closed (TUR) surgery, too. The shaving is usually performed on the evening before or on the day of surgery; it may be uncomfortable, but it is not painful.

ANESTHESIA

Except in emergencies, the anesthesiologist meets the patient before surgery, giving both of them an opportunity to discuss any concerns and to make the final decision regarding the type of anesthesia to use.

There are several types of anesthesia, and not all are appropriate for every kind of surgery. *Topical anesthesia* is sprayed or painted on an area and offers only superficial numbing. *Local anesthesia* is injected into the surgical site, completely numbing the area; this is used mostly for minor procedures. *Regional anesthesia* is similar to local anesthesia, except that it affects a much larger area. *Spinal anesthesia* involves the injection of a drug into the sac that surrounds the spinal cord, which is part of the central nervous system. The result is a complete loss of feeling in the legs and much of the lower part of the body. This effect lingers for several hours following surgery, and the patient feels some discomfort when it wears off. A person is sedated prior to spinal anesthesia.

General anesthesia is administered intravenously, by inhalation, or by a combination of both. Intravenous anesthesia goes directly into the bloodstream; inhalation anesthesia consists of gases that are breathed through a mask and travel through the lungs into the bloodstream.

Most urologists prefer spinal anesthesia to general anesthesia for prostate surgery. This is because postoperative bleeding is increased in patients awakening from general anesthesia as they strain to cough.

BLOOD TRANSFUSIONS

During any of the procedures for prostatectomy, blood transfusions may be needed. Unless the patient is a member of a blood program that offers free blood replacement, he might wish to ask family and friends to donate blood for him. Blood is expensive, and many insurance policies (Medicare included) do *not* pay for the first few pints.

Since most communities occasionally or even frequently experience a shortage in their blood supplies, asking friends for donations of a pint of blood in lieu of flowers or cookies is also a fine way to help bolster the supply. Some hospitals, such as the Mount Sinai Medical Center in New York City, allow "directed donors." Thus, people can donate blood and state that it is to be saved for a specific patient; if it turns out not to be needed by that patient, it may be made available to someone who does need it.

All blood today, whether from strangers, friends, or family, is carefully screened for hepatitis, AIDS, and other diseases that can be transferred by blood products. Still, a patient may wish to donate his own blood in advance of the surgery. This procedure allows what is called an *autologous transfusion*. A person can give blood for his own future use up to thirty-five days prior to the surgery during which it will be needed. Blood can be stored for longer periods if it is frozen, but freezing blood is expensive, and not all hospitals have the facilities for doing it. When freezing blood is not done at the hospital blood bank, it may be possible to make arrangements with a private laboratory that will then transport the blood to the hospital prior to the patient's surgery.

Gail Button, RN, of the Mount Sinai Medical Center Blood Bank, says that the ideal time for a donor-recipient to come into the blood bank is three weeks prior to surgery. This enables the patient to recover fully from the donation, and it allows the blood to remain fresh for use if needed during surgery or in the week following surgery.

Blood used during prostate surgery is composed of packed cells; the blood type must be compatible with the patient's blood type, but it need not match.

TRANSURETHRAL RESECTION (TUR)

If the prostate is not exceedingly large (50 to 60 grams and sometimes larger), most urologists will perform a transurethral resection (TUR). In this procedure, the doctor is usually able to remove as much of the prostate tissue from the capsule as he would have been able to remove if he had begun with an incision. Sometimes only part of the gland has to be removed to afford the patient relief from his symptoms. This is the procedure that President Ronald Reagan underwent in January 1987, when a urologist removed 23.5 grams of his prostatic tissue.

The first step in the TUR procedure is the insertion of a nonflexible synthetic hollow tube into the penis and urethra. Through this tube passes the sophisticated transurethral fiber optic microlens system, more commonly known as a resectoscope. One of the functions of this system is to provide complete illumination of the field, clearly showing the obstruction. The urologist can see inside the bladder as clearly as you might see the inside of the stadium at a night ballgame.

The urologist then slips an electric loop through the hollow tube and moves it back and forth to cut away prostatic tissue. A foot pedal activates the electrical power, leaving the urologist's hands free for the surgery. A second foot pedal operates a coagulating device through the same loop; when the loop is placed over a bleeding area and the coagulating pedal is pressed, the device seals off the open blood vessel. As he works, the surgeon constantly observes the entire area through a lens located just outside the penis. Glycine (a fluid) constantly irrigates the urethra while the surgery is in progress. The prostatic tissue is removed in the form of shavings or chips, and this tissue is studied by a pathologist after the operation to determine if cancer is present.

Removing all or most of the prostate creates a good urinary canal. The surgical capsule (the shell) is exposed but not removed. A catheter (a thin, smooth, flexible hollow tube, made of rubber or plastic) is then passed through the penis and the urethra and into the bladder, to draw urine directly from the bladder. It remains in place for a few days because of bleeding. After it is removed, the patient is again able to urinate naturally.

The catheter inserted after a TUR usually has three openings: one to allow fluid to go in; one to allow fluid to come out; and a third, with an inflatable balloon at the end, to keep the catheter from falling out. Through the catheter, a stream of saline solution (water and salt) is introduced to irrigate and cleanse the bladder. This saline solution usually remains in circulation for about twenty-four hours; the catheter to drain urine from the bladder remains in place for an additional two or three days. The hospital staff remind the patient to drink plenty of fluids as a natural way to flush and cleanse his system. Most patients are helped out of bed within twenty-four hours after surgery and should be feeling quite well within a few days. The patient can walk around with the catheter in place; it is a bit awkward, but not uncomfortable.

When the catheter is removed (usually on the third or fourth day after surgery), the patient will be able to urinate comfortably by himself. There is no need to worry that removal of the catheter will be painful; when the balloon of the catheter is deflated, the catheter simply slides out by itself when the patient stands up. The next day, the patient can go home.

Occasionally a patient is unable to urinate comfortably on his own. It may be that his urethra is taking a little longer than expected to heal, or he may simply be frightened about trying to urinate. Many people, regardless of the kind of surgery they have, are afraid to urinate or to move their bowels after surgery. Knowing that he is not alone in experiencing this anxiety may be all the reassurance a patient needs in order to take this next step toward independence.

If urination remains a problem, the catheter will be reinserted. A local anesthetic preparation such as Xylocaine can be instilled (in a measured volume) in the urethra through the penis to eliminate any discomfort during reinsertion of the catheter. (If the doctor should try to insert a catheter without medication, the patient has every right to question him.)

If all goes according to schedule, the patient will probably go home on the fourth, fifth, or sixth day after admission to the hospital. (If there is a delay of a few days, it will not lessen the totality of the recovery.)

The departing patient may be given a prescription for an antibiotic to be taken orally for two to four weeks, to prevent any possible infection or inflammation. He may be advised to take hot sitz baths, rather than showers, to help reduce inflammation and congestion at the operative site. He will also be told to drink plenty of liquids, to avoid spicy foods, and to take precautions (for example, using a mild laxative or eating sensibly) to avoid becoming constipated. Although there will be some limits on his activity, a post-TUR patient usually finds that he can get back to his normal routine fairly quickly, including driving a car. He may have some slight burning or discomfort during the first week or two when he urinates, and he may even find some blood in his urine during the first three months back at home. This is not cause for serious alarm, but the patient should tell his urologist, who may decide to help control the situation with medication.

The urologist will probably want to see the recovering patient a week or two after discharge, and again every few months thereafter. At some point, the urologist may want the patient to have a sonogram or x-ray, and may continue to monitor him yearly.

A person whose job allows him to sit at a desk most of the time can go back to work about two or three weeks after surgery. A man who must stay on his feet a lot, however, will be more comfortable if he waits a little longer before returning to work.

A person who does moderately heavy work—a truck driver, for example—should plan on being away from the job for three to four weeks, and someone who does very heavy labor should allow himself a month to six weeks before going back to work. Of course, age and physical condition prior to surgery, as well as individual recuperative abilities, may alter this timetable.

Regardless of how well he is feeling, the patient will be advised to abstain from sexual activity for at least six weeks after the operation, to allow for full healing and to avoid bleeding.

TUR VERSUS OPEN SURGERY

A TUR is the simplest operation for BPH, and most urologists would prefer to perform it because initial recovery from the operation is faster than with open surgery; however, the full recovery period is the same.

Many years ago, some urologists did *only* TURs. An interesting bit of history will shed some light on the reason behind this. In the late 1920s and early 1930s, urology was not recognized as a specialty at the famed Mayo Clinic in Minnesota. Consequently, prostatectomy (open prostate surgery) came under the heading of general surgery, and Drs. Charles and William Mayo refused to allow urologists to perform such surgery. Urologists were, however, allowed to perform TURs—but only if the prostate's size was graded at 1 or 2 (the two smaller sizes), rather than at 3 or 4 (the two larger sizes). Faced with these limitations on his area of practice, a very competent urologist on the Mayo Clinic staff named Dr. H. Carey Bumpus simply identified all prostates in need of surgery as either grade 1 or grade 2, and performed TURs on them.

When Dr. Bumpus worked with the Greenberger associates in New York City in the early 1930s, he learned to do open surgery, which most urologists in the east were already using for greatly enlarged prostates. The doctors in the east were impressed with the competence with which Dr. Bumpus was able to remove giant prostates transurethrally. But today if a urologist tells a patient that he only does TURs, the patient should find himself another doctor!

Most urologists feel that if a man's prostate is so enlarged that they cannot easily remove virtually the entire gland by means of a TUR within 1 to 1½ hours, they would rather perform open surgery. If the patient is in his sixties, is in fairly good health, and has a large prostate, the chances are good that he will be back in five, ten, or even twenty years with the same symptoms if an incomplete TUR is performed. Interestingly, President Ronald Reagan had a TUR performed twenty years prior to the one that gained national attention in 1987. Many men—unlike the energetic president—find that twenty years later they are not only older but considerably less healthy and less prepared to deal with another surgical procedure. This potential problem can usually (but not always) be avoided if the entire prostate tissue is removed the first time, either by TUR or by open surgery. When treating an older man or one in poor health, urologists sometimes compromise and do a partial TUR; this affords him comfort, and minimizes any risks.

To remove all of the prostate, urologists are trained to perform two procedures in addition to TUR: the suprapubic prostatectomy and the retropubic prostatectomy. Although some urologists prefer one over the other, most perform the one that is more clearly indicated in a given situation.

Sometimes a urologist cannot decide before surgery if he will be able to perform a TUR or must resort to one of the types of the open surgery. This happens when the prostate is a borderline size—usually somewhere around 60 grams. Occasionally, when the patient is already in the operating room, the urologist finds he cannot insert the instrument for the TUR because of a stricture in the urethra. To deal with this problem, the urologist dilates the urethra by inserting (and then removing) a thin metal instrument through the penis and urethra, stretching the urethra. Then, either at the same time or at a later date, the urologist performs a TUR.

SUPRAPUBIC PROSTATECTOMY

In a suprapubic prostatectomy, a vertical incision may be made from a point below the navel to a point just above the pubis (the first bone below the navel) in the lower abdomen, or a horizontal incision may be made above the pubic hair. Depending on the man's size, the incision is about 4 to 6 inches long. The incision is made through the skin and its lining, the fascia. The muscles covering the bladder are separated, the peritoneum (the closed membranous sac covering the entire abdominal wall of the body) is retracted (pulled back), and an incision is made into the bladder. The surgeon can then see if there are any stones, tumors, or diverticuli (out-pouchings) in the bladder—any of which can easily be removed if necessary. Next, the prostate gland (also clearly visible) is removed. As in a TUR, the tissue is examined to ascertain whether cancer is present. If a bladder tumor is suspected as a result of preoperative tests, a cystoscopy is performed just before surgery.

All bleeding vessels are sutured or cauterized; the stitches dissolve by themselves after surgery. After all the bleeding is controlled, a catheter is passed through the penis and into the bladder to irrigate it and to empty it. Just before the bladder is closed by the surgeon, a second (called a suprapubic catheter) is inserted directly into the bladder, passing through the muscle fascia and skin, and emerging just below the umbilicus. Its purpose is to keep the bladder empty of urine *and* irrigating fluid and because it is larger than the one that goes through the penis, it more effectively drains the bladder during the post-operative period.

The process of continuous irrigation is usually discontinued in one or two days, and the suprapubic catheter is removed the next day. The catheter that passes through the penis remains in place for six or seven days after surgery, to remove urine from the bladder and to permit normal healing. When it is removed, the patient is usually able to urinate on his own and returns home the next day. If he has trouble urinating, the catheter is reinserted, after a local anesthetic preparation is instilled—just as may happen after a TUR—and he is allowed another day or two for healing before another urination trial is given and the patient is discharged from the hospital.

RETROPUBIC PROSTATECTOMY

The same incision is made in a retropubic prostatectomy as in a suprapubic one. The incision is made through the skin and the fascia, the muscle is separated, and the peritoneum containing the intestines is pushed away from the bladder. Instead of opening the bladder, however, the surgeon makes an incision into the prostatic capsule and removes the gland. This tissue is subjected to testing to make sure that cancer is not present. After the prostate is removed, all bleeding vessels are sutured, and a three-way catheter is passed through the penis and the capsule, and into the bladder. This three-way catheter is identical to the one used in a TUR. The balloon is inflated, the capsule is sutured closed, and the muscle, fascia, and skin are also tightly closed.

In this procedure, because the bladder is left closed, there is no need to drain the bladder with a suprapubic catheter. All the draining and irrigation can be done through the three-way catheter. This method takes about the same amount of time to execute as a suprapubic prostatectomy, but often it seems to be less stressful to the patient, because the bladder is not cut and there is only one tube in the bladder. But there is essentially no difference in the length of the recovery period. Many urologists who use both methods find it difficult to explain why they prefer one over the other. The retropubic is a bit more difficult in obese patients because the doctor has to work in a small space. Consequently, many urologists prefer to do suprapubic prostatectomies on obese patients. With thin or medium-built individuals, however, they might choose to do either retropubic or suprapubic prostatectomies.

Patients who have had either a suprapubic or a retropubic prostatectomy can expect to go home around eight days after surgery. They can bathe and shower immediately, usually resume driving a week or two later, and return to work within the next few weeks. Just as in recuperations after TURs, men whose occupations require heavy labor must wait longer to return to work than men who do sedentary work. About six weeks after surgery, a man can do anything he did before surgery—including have sex. There is no reason to anticipate that the patient will have any problems with sex following surgery for BPH (unless, of course, he had sexual problems prior to his prostate trouble).

PERINEAL PROSTATECTOMY

A third open surgical procedure, called a perineal prostatectomy, is almost never performed anymore. In this procedure, an incision is made through the perineum (the area between the anal opening and the scrotum), and the prostate is removed through that incision. This is a direct route to the prostate and may sound like a good idea, but it almost always severs nerves and leaves the patient impotent. Stricture formation, which resembles and behaves like scar tissue, often occurs too.

Stricture formation can follow any of the surgical procedures described, but the Greenberger associates (who in their early years did quite a few perineal prostatectomies) found that it was much more frequent with the perineal approach than with any other. A man who develops stricture formation in the urethra (signaled by a thin, narrow urinary stream) can be dilated in the office a few times to help relieve the resulting discomfort in urinating. Of course, just as before inserting a catheter or cystoscope used for dilation, the urologist instills some Xylocaine or other local anesthetic to make the procedure painless. Without dilation, the patient will continue to suffer much the same discomfort he felt prior to surgery.

Years ago, the perineal approach was perceived as offering some advantages because it afforded the urologist a good view of the rear of the prostate, which is where cancer often exists. But examination prior to surgery usually informs the doctor if cancer is or may be present, and sonograms, x-rays, and laboratory tests (the pathology report) on the tissue removed during a biopsy or surgery will settle any such question. A proponent of the perineal approach may also argue that this procedure leaves little postoperative discomfort and that recovery is rapid, so that it is a good method for the older patient who does not mind being left impotent. But how many men of any age are willing to be rendered impotent, if there is an alternative treatment available—even if they are not sexually active at the time? Thus, the perineal approach was abandoned long ago by most urologists. If a urologist suggests performing this particular operation, the patient would be wise to seek another opinion.

NEW SURGICAL APPROACHES

In some medical centers, urologists are attempting a new method of surgically treating BPH by cryosurgery. This technique involves inserting a probe that contains liquid nitrogen through the penis and urethra and into the prostate. The probe is then used to shrink away swollen tissue. Other urologists are trying laser surgery. But as of 1987 and 1988 many urologists were not enthusiastic about these methods for treating BPH, although they say that these procedures may become valuable in the future, possibly for treating cancer of the prostate.

OLD AND MODERN TWO-STAGE PROCEDURES

Doctors used to perform a two-stage procedure almost exclusively, back in the 1920s and early 1930s. The first stage in that procedure consisted of draining the bladder by making a 4- to 6-inch opening below the umbilicus. A tube was then placed in the bladder to allow drainage of urine. Some time between seven and fourteen days afterward, the second stage began. An incision was made through the skin, muscle, and bladder, and the prostate was removed. Packing was then placed in the prostatic cavity (the area from which the prostate had been removed), and then the bladder, muscle, and skin were closed around another drainage tube. In about two to five days, the packing was removed. Each of these three steps required general or spinal anesthesia. The patient remained in the hospital another few weeks after the third step was completed.

This procedure is not done today, but a modern version, cystostomy, is still practiced in instances of "silent prostatism"—especially if a patient has almost developed uremia (with kidney function affected) or if the patient has some unrelated medical problems and needs to wait until these conditions improve before undergoing prostatectomy.

In the modern cystostomy, the tube is first placed in the bladder as described earlier. This is actually a rather simple procedure. Often it is done with a simple punch, rather than with an incision.

A person who has this procedure done usually goes home after drainage has begun and he is medically stable; he then returns to the hospital in one to nine months for the second stage. While at home between stages of surgery, the patient wears a leg bag, which collects urine coming from the tube in the bladder. The patient can easily learn to care for the tube and bag himself, removing it in order to take a tub bath or shower. During the period at home, he will not be bedridden nor limited in most of his activities. It is even possible for him to go back to work. He can exercise by walking or playing golf; he can also drive a car, travel, have sexual relations, and do whatever else he could do before surgery.

After the second stage of the surgical procedure, when the prostate is actually removed, the patient can again urinate on his own, and the remainder of the recovery should be uneventful.

Obviously, no particular operation is perfect for everyone who has BPH. Instead, the procedure chosen depends on a combination of factors, including the extent of prostatic enlargement and the patient's age and general health. The urologist's own particular preference is also important, and it should be respected, provided that he is willing and able to perform whichever procedure is most appropriate to the case.

SIMULTANEOUS PROCEDURES

Surgery to correct other problems is not usually performed at the same time as BPH, although certain conditions in the urinary tract might be handled simultaneously. If there is a diverticulum of the bladder (an outpouching), it can be removed when a suprapubic prostatectomy is performed. If there are stones in the bladder, they can also be removed.

AFTER SURGERY

After any kind of surgery the patient will probably be removed to a recovery room, and then, in some hospitals, to a surgical intensive-care unit. When his condition seems stable, he will be moved back to his own room. The timetable for this varies widely, so family and friends should not worry about how soon the patient returns to his own room.

FINAL RECOVERY

Understanding in advance the procedures involved in removing the prostate usually helps alleviate a man's presurgical fears. Patients usually find that some of their apprehension is put to rest during the initial office visit, when they learn that nothing will be inserted into the penis without local anesthetic being instilled first. Most patents are so miserable with their symptoms of BPH that they are eager for relief; and relief is what they get, although some minor symptoms may persist temporarily until complete healing takes place. For example, at first a man may still feel the urgent need to urinate frequently, and his urinary stream may still be weak. He *may* also have some urinary leakage, occasional bladder spasms (mild contractions), or some bleeding that causes a slight discoloration of urine. These symptoms are not inevitable and are not reason for worry, since they should improve with time. A patient should discuss any such concerns with his urologist.

Most men experience a vast improvement—if not immediately, soon. Hesitancy, straining to void, the sensation of incomplete bladder emptying, and dribbling of urine will be relieved. Some older men continue to experience frequency and are still awakened during the night by the need to urinate. Generally, those symptoms persist because the bladder itself has aged, but they are not due to incomplete emptying and therefore do not lead to kidney damage. Because a man feels better generally, his sexual functioning may even be improved, so that life really can begin anew after the surgery. Within a few months, the prostate trouble seems a distant memory. In fact, the recovered patient might even forget to go back for checkups if he does not mark it on his calendar or if his urologist does not send him a reminder to do so!

7

CANCER OF THE PROSTATE

Even after many years of practice, most physicians still get a heavy feeling in their hearts when they have to tell a patient that he has cancer. But today they are also able to tell him that the prognosis for men who have cancer of the prostate is considerably brighter than it was years ago.

Many people shudder at hearing the word *cancer*. To them, it is synonymous with death. But if they understood cancer better, they would know that it often can be treated successfully, and that many healthy, pain-free, and comfortable years may still lie before them. In cancer, more even than in other diseases, early detection is extremely important for successful treatment.

Cancer, quite simply, is an uncontrolled growth of abnormal cells. Unlike BPH, where the gland grows and may crowd the urethra but does not spread to other parts of the body, cancer cells can spread around (metastasize) and replace normal tissue. The cancerous cells form tumors and tend to spread through the blood or lymph system to other parts of the body, where they create "new" tumors.

Cancer cells may spread in an orderly fashion, or they may spread chaotically. A cancerous tumor that originates in one part of the body may show up almost immediately or much later in a distant area. When cancer is discovered very early (while it is still contained in one place), however, it can often be cured. Although doctors use the word *cure* cautiously, preferring the phrase "no evidence of disease," the reality is that some cancers, such as prostate cancer, can be cured under certain circumstances. But even when a complete cure is not possible, surgery, radiation, hormones, or chemotherapy may render the cancer inactive or dormant for many years—perhaps for a natural lifetime.

Cancer of the prostate is almost always a primary cancer; that is, it originates in that site, rather than traveling from other parts of the body to the prostate, although some cancers may travel to areas close to the prostate. If cancer of the prostate is left untreated, it can spread through and out of the prostate capsule and eventually metastasize through the lymph system to the bones, lungs, chest, and even brain.

INCIDENCE

The American Cancer Society estimates that about one out of every eleven men will develop cancer of the prostate at some time in his lifetime. Approximately 96,000 cases were diagnosed in the United States in 1987. Excluding nonmelanoma skin cancer, prostate cancer is the second most common cancer in men, just behind lung cancer.

Prostate cancer is age-related: cancer of the prostate is rare in men under the age of fifty, and the average age of men at the time of diagnosis is seventy-three. About 80 percent of all prostate cancers are discovered in men who are over the age of sixty-five. It is so common that, according to many reliable estimates, by age eighty almost all men have some beginnings of it. It is not always diagnosed, however, and many men in their eighties will never have any symptoms and will die of unrelated causes.

An estimated 27,000 men die of prostate cancer each year. This number could be considerably lowered if the diagnoses were made earlier, since a simple digital rectal examination can uncover many early cases. At present, only 63 percent of all prostate cancers are discovered while they are still limited to the prostate as a small nodule; the survival rate for men who are treated at this early stage is high (83 percent of such men are alive five years after treatment), and it is steadily increasing. During the last twenty years, according to the American Cancer Society, five-year survival rates for all patients with cancer of the prostate, including those diagnosed after the cancer had spread, has increased from 48 percent to 70 percent.

But because so many cases of prostate cancer are diagnosed *after* they have begun to spread, it remains the third-highest cause of cancer deaths in men aged fifty-five to seventy-four, exceeded only by lung cancer and colon and rectal cancer. Among men aged seventy-five and over, it is the second-highest cause of cancer deaths in men, following lung cancer. Despite this high incidence, prostatic cancer accounts for only 10 percent of all cancer deaths in men, as compared to 36 percent caused by lung cancer.

Because cancer of the prostate is almost exclusively a disease of older men, its occurrence has been on the rise as increasing numbers of men live long enough to develop the disease. When diagnosed and treated early on in a man of *any* age, it can have a good prognosis. In men over the age of seventy, cancer tends to grow extremely slowly, as has been proved in major university studies. No wonder the Greenberger files are full of case histories

81

of men who were treated for cancer of the prostate and went on to live full and cancer-free lives. These men usually had a personal physician who was a strong advocate of regular digital rectal examinations and who sent them to a urologist promptly if anything suspect was found.

CAUSES AND RISK FACTORS

The cause of cancer of the prostate is unknown. It is a disease found almost exclusively in human beings—which, of course, prevents meaningful experiments in animals. No clear evidence links smoking, drinking, diet, viral infections, venereal disease, occupational exposure (except among men who work in the presence of automobile exhaust fumes or cadmium, who are found to be at a slightly higher risk), or environmental factors to the development of prostatic cancer. Many studies have produced conflicting results; for instance, some studies suggest that men who have had a large number of sexual partners or a prior history of venereal disease are at greater risk, but other studies suggest that men who have little or no sexual outlet are at greater risk.

Although the causes of prostate cancer are still unknown, statistical evidence suggests that the incidence and mortality of prostate cancer among blacks is twice that among whites. The rate is higher in Northwest Europe and North America than in the Orient and Eastern Europe. There may be some tendencies in families to develop prostate cancer, but researchers do not know whether these are the result of genetic or environmental causes. Years ago, the incidence of prostate cancer was unusually low in Americans of Asian extraction; the reasons for this are not fully understood, although they may be both genetically and environmentally related (to diet, in particular). Studies indicate that the gap is gradually closing. Occasionally, studies conclude that men with low-cholesterol diets—as well as those who are vegetarians or eat a great many green and yellow vegetables—have relatively low rates of prostatic cancer.

IMPORTANCE OF EARLY DETECTION

Cancer of the prostate usually originates in the periphery of the gland, beneath the capsule. If a man's personal physician feels a stony, hard mass or nodule of any size during a normal rectal digital examination, he will suspect cancer and will send him to a urologist for a more definitive diagnosis.

Regular rectal examinations of the prostate are as vital for men as Pap smears and breast examinations are for women. Many famous women, from movie stars to presidents' wives, have discussed their experiences with breast cancer; and the information media remind women that mammograms and breast self-examination are crucial to early detection. Comparatively little attention, however, has been paid to prostate cancer detection.

Rose Kushner, a prominent consumer advocate for women with breast cancer, has publicly pleaded for some male celebrity to step forward and tell the world that he has had prostate cancer and that, because it was discovered early, his personal (including sexual) life and his work life are continuing uninterrupted. Too many men are fearful of discovering that they have cancer of the prostate because they fear a loss of sexual functioning. In the present day, that fear has far less grounds in reality than it once had.

IS IT CANCER?

A diagnosis of prostatic cancer can be reached in any of several ways: by rectal examination, by examination of tissue from the prostate, by visualization techniques (sonograms, x-rays, and so on), and by various blood tests. If cancer is found to be present, the urologist will perform a number of additional tests to establish whether the cancer is still entirely contained within the prostate or has spread. Because the malignancy usually originates in a part of the prostate that does not cause urinary obstruction, early prostate cancer is seldom accompanied by any of the obvious symptoms a man might experience in prostatitis or BPH. Frequently, however (especially in older men), cancer of the prostate and BPH coexist, but these two conditions are unrelated.

After an operation for BPH, such as a TUR, the routine pathological examination of the prostatic tissue sometimes reveals malignant cells in the gland. Cancer discovered in this way is probably at such an early stage that less than 5 percent of the total glandular involvement is cancerous. It may consist of only a few chips of removed tissue, so that a rectal examination conducted by even a highly trained and skilled urologist would not have discovered it. When this happens, a patient is more fully evaluated to determine if any special treatment is indicated.

Sometimes weight loss, shortness of breath, symptoms of illness, or pain in the pelvis, lower back, or upper thighs first sends a man to his personal physician. These symptoms may signify nothing serious at all, or they may be associated with cancer of the prostate that has spread throughout the capsule and into adjacent lymph nodes or bones.

DIAGNOSTIC STEPS

When a urologist conducts the digital rectal examination and feels a hard nodule, he will want to have some of the tissue examined to determine whether or not it is cancerous. Until recently, he had little choice: he did a biopsy, using a needle inserted through the rectum or perineum to remove a core of tissue. This procedure, which is done in the office or in the out-patient department of a hospital, requires a local anesthesia and is sometimes associated with bleeding or (in the case of the transrectal biopsy) with infection. But now a newer method is employed by many urologists. Called *fine-needle aspiration cytology,* it is a quick, safe, and excellent diagnostic technique. (Aspiration is the removal of fluid or tissue by suction.) Urologists who are experienced with the technique describe it as a simple, relatively painless (no anesthesia is needed), three-minute office procedure in which the urologist inserts a very fine needle through the patient's rectum and removes cells from approximately four different spots in the prostate. The risks of bleeding and infection are minimal. Occasionally, if the cytology (examination of cells or tissue) report is dubious, a urologist will repeat the aspiration or perform the more traditional biopsy of the prostate, in order to get a larger sample of tissue.

If the biopsy indicates cancer, further tests are conducted to find out the extent of the cancer and to allow for planning of appropriate treatment. If the biopsy is negative for cancer, but the urologist remains suspicious as a result of his digital examination, he may repeat the biopsy in a few months.

Two blood tests performed prior to biopsy provide information regarding the possibility of cancer in the prostate. These are the prostatic acid phosphatase (PAP) test and the prostate specific antigen (PSA) test. An elevated PAP suggests that prostatic cancer has spread; the PSA indicates the probability of prostatic cancer. These elevations can also occur, however, if a man has been examined rectally and the prostate has been massaged even slightly, because the PAP and PSA may then travel from their natural habitat (the prostate) into the bloodstream. Thus, blood drawn from a man within twenty-four hours after a rectal examination will show an elevation of this enzyme that has no connection whatsoever to cancer of the prostate. Conversely, the disease may metastasize and yet not cause an elevated acid phosphatase level; and it can exist without causing the PSA to be elevated, either. Obviously, these tests must be corroborated by other tests, but they do alert the doctor to look further. The tests are also used in the course of later treatment to monitor the patient's response to the treatment program.

Radioimmunoassay, an excellent, sensitive analytical technique, is used to measure substances present in the blood in amounts too small to be detected by other methods. Thus, it can spot the most minute increase in the blood's PAP or PSA level and so suggest the presence of even local disease. Some physicians have suggested that the use of PAP, PSA, and radioimmunoassay techniques may eventually be used for mass screening of prostate cancer, just as the Pap (short for *Papanicolaou*) smear is used for early detection of cervical cancer in women. Over and over, however, the most prominent urologists at major medical schools say that the digital rectal examination remains the best diagnostic tool for discovering cancer.

To determine if cancer of the prostate has spread, the urologist may order a number of imaging tests. In all likelihood, he will order chest x-rays, bone scans, and

CAT scans of the abdomen and of the entire pelvic area. He will want to know if the cancer has spread to the seminal vesicles, so he may order a transrectal sonogram as well as the abdominal scan, if necessary.

The urologist may want to perform a biopsy of the lymph nodes surrounding the prostatic area. This is a surgical procedure called a *pelvic lymphadenectomy,* and it is sometimes used to determine the presence or absence of metastatic tumors in the pelvic lymph nodes. The urologist may also want a pedal lymphangiogram performed, in which dye is injected between the first and second and between the second and third toes of each foot, in order to stain the lymphatic vessels. As the dye moves through the body, films are taken of the abdomen, pelvis, and upper body. Aspiration of suspicious nodes may also be performed.

In most instances, all of these tests are conducted before treatment begins; but if the prostate cancer was discovered during surgery for BPH, the tests will be performed afterward to determine if the cancer was indeed limited to the small area of the prostate.

DETERMINING THE APPROPRIATE TREATMENT

Most cancers are described by reference to a universally agreed upon series of stages, but some discrepancies still exist in the way prostate cancer is described. Moreover, total agreement on treatment for each stage does not exist. Treatments that have been demonstrated to be successful will be described here—but every patient should understand that the urologist will plan the course of his treatment on the basis of many factors, including the extent of the disease, the patient's general health, and the patient's age. In many instances, where more than one treatment has proved valuable, the patient may be given a choice. As in all medical matters, patients certainly should consider getting a second opinion.

When prostate cancer is confined to the prostate, cure is the goal of treatment. Surgical removal of the prostate is a method advocated by a good number of urologists. Radiotherapy—either externally directed or generated by radioactive material that has been implanted into the prostate—is another method that has many proponents. Because statistics prove that, in men over the age of seventy, the prostate cancer is likely to grow very slowly, some urologists do not recommend treatment of older men if no spread of the cancer has occurred at time of diagnosis. For instance, if a man has had a TUR during which only a single focus or a few chips of cancer were found in the gland, and if no further cancer seems to remain (upon digital examination or the conducting of a sonogram), it seems unlikely that his cancer will progress. Many urologists believe that the man can be well served by being watched carefully with regular examinations, blood tests, sonograms, and bone scans.

Other urologists argue that they can never be absolutely certain that every single cancer cell has been removed; therefore, since 20 to 25 percent of men will experience progress of cancer during the ensuing ten- to fifteen-year period, they assert that such a man deserves to have his body rid of the cancer with some certainty.

When several urologists were asked what they would recommend if a patient of seventy-two with this localized cancer happened to be their brother or father—or themselves—most of them quoted statistics that indicate that a man of that age is more likely to die of some other disease before the untreated prostate cancer causes his demise. But when pressed for an answer as to what they would recommend to a cherished individual patient, they tended to give answers that assumed a more personal tone. The physicians recognized that an otherwise healthy, active man of seventy-two could possibly— against all so-called statistics—live another ten or twenty productive years, and they felt that he should be given the opportunity to be treated in a manner that increases the likelihood of a cure. Thus, a urologist should explain all of the various options to the patient, who can then make his own decision.

If the cancer has spread beyond the prostate, a man of any age will benefit from treatment, which can allow him to enjoy a number of healthy, pain-free years. Such treatment is usually based on findings that go back to 1941, when Dr. Charles Huggins introduced the concept of reducing the quantity of male hormones in the patient in order to treat cancer of the prostate. This may be accomplished surgically or by administering female hormones, as described on pages 91–92 and 97–99.

STANDARD SURGICAL TREATMENTS

Since the turn of the century, urologists have known that the only way to effect a total cure in a man whose prostate cancer had not spread beyond the capsule was to remove the entire prostate and capsule in a procedure called *radical prostatectomy*. Nonetheless, they often hesitated to recommend this procedure, because almost 90 percent of all men who underwent such surgery were left sexually impotent. The reason for this is that nerves lying close to the prostate and controlling erection were cut during the standard radical surgical procedures. Urologists noted, however, that some patients remained potent after surgery, and this led to investigation of how to perform this surgery so as to avoid its highly undesirable side effect.

Patrick Walsh, M.D., director of the Department of Urology at the Johns Hopkins University School of Medicine, after conducting painstaking research, identified the two neurovascular bundles of nerves that controlled erection and devised a procedure that enabled surgeons to remove the prostate and capsule while sparing these nerves. Even if one bundle is cut or damaged during surgery, potency can be preserved. This nerve-sparing surgery uses the same retropubic approach previously discussed in relation to surgery for BPH. In this procedure, a horizontal or vertical incision is made through the skin and fascia below the navel, and then the prostate and capsule are removed. The patient's recovery and convalescent period is similar to that following surgery for BPH: a three-way catheter is inserted into his bladder (through the penis and urethra) to allow irrigation and drainage of urine until healing has taken place; then, within a week or two, he will be home—free of cancer. His health will, of course, be monitored closely by the urologist, who will do frequent blood tests, sonograms, and bone scans to make sure that no stray cancer cells are left to spread.

Although patients who undergo the nerve-sparing radical prostatectomy developed by Dr. Walsh are not immediately potent (because nerves are sometimes damaged and need time to heal), 70 percent of them gradually (over the next year or two) regain the ability to achieve an erection sufficient for penetration. The success rate is greatest among younger patients (probably for reasons related to overall function) and among those with the least amount of tumor.

Increasing numbers of urologists can do this surgery, and as Michael Droller, M.D., chairman of the Department of Urology at the Mount Sinai School of Medicine in New York, says, "Physicians should keep themselves updated and be familiar with this technique, but if a urologist has not yet mastered it, he should say, 'I don't do it but I will refer you to someone who does do it.' " Dr. Droller feels that patients should feel comfortable asking a urologist if he will do this new nerve-sparing procedure for cancer of the prostate, rather than undergoing the older procedure that almost always results in impotence. Under Dr. Droller's leadership, the urologists at Mount Sinai all perform this procedure, and patients should be able to find a similarly trained urologist at any large teaching hospital.

Patients sometimes ask whether this procedure provides as high a level of cancer control and cure as the old surgery did. All studies conducted thus far indicate that it does.

If the cancer has spread, a radical prostatectomy is not advised by urologists today. Instead, they may suggest any of various treatments, including the surgery introduced and first described by Dr. Charles Huggins in Chicago at a 1941 meeting of the American Urological Association. The Greenberger associates heard his presentation at this meeting and, upon returning to New York City, became among the first doctors there to perform this procedure, called a *bilateral orchiectomy* (removal of both testicles, leaving the scrotal bag intact). Some of the patients treated with this surgery in the 1940s lived on for a long time and eventually died of unrelated causes.

In this procedure, impotence is likely to follow, and sterility is a certainty; but some of the other fears of men can be allayed. For instance, the removal of the testicles is not evident, since the scrotum remains. Indeed, if a man so desires, the scrotum can be filled with a synthetic substance, so that the outward appearance remains exactly the same as it was prior to surgery.

The purpose underlying a bilateral orchiectomy is to remove the male hormones (most of which are manufactured in the testes), in order to inhibit the growth of the prostate cancer. Although this surgical procedure does not cure prostate cancer, it can keep the cancer at bay for some twenty years. Is it any wonder that many urologists still recommend this surgery to men, despite the side effects?

Urologists differ in their judgment as to what stage of the disease is appropriate for treatment with a bilateral orchiectomy. Some suggest it at first detection of the onset of a spread, while others prefer to wait until the symptoms of metastasis are pronounced. It is *not* recommended for treatment of cancer that is wholly confined to the prostate.

Despite its effectiveness, many men refuse this surgery. Many men imagine that they will be turned into eunuchs with high soprano voices and no facial hair, not realizing that these features are the result of castration before puberty. For a man who has had a full quota of male hormones throughout his life, the results of bilateral orchiectomy should not noticeably affect his voice, appearance, or personality. Still, it is a matter that should be frankly and carefully discussed between patient and doctor. It is, of course, a decision that the patient must make, but he should be aware that most men opt for the treatment that offers them the best overall quality of life—even if it limits their sexual functioning. As is discussed in chapter 9, it is often possible for a man to have a penile prosthesis inserted that allows him to have an erection that he would otherwise be unable to achieve.

CRYOSURGERY AND LASER SURGERY

Cryosurgery, as a treatment for cancer of the prostate, involves inserting a probe cooled to a very low temperature into the prostate, where (theoretically) it freezes and destroys the cancer.

Laser surgery, which makes use of an extremely concentrated beam of light waves and particles that emits sufficient heat to destroy anything in its path, may someday play a role in the treatment of cancer of the prostate. At present, however, these modalities are still highly experimental.

RADIATION THERAPY

Radiation is electromagnetic energy emitted from some source in the form of rays that can pass through certain substances, including skin and flesh. *Radiation therapy* (also known as *radiotherapy* or *x-ray therapy*) is a general term used to describe the use of these rays to slow or halt the growth of cancer cells or to destroy such cells. It is very effective in curing prostate cancer; consequently, it is often used in place of surgery to treat cancer that is limited to the prostate.

Radiation therapy has come a long way since its introduction in the 1920s and 1930s, when x-ray machines operated on low power and caused many side effects on the skin and throughout the body. Today's megavolt or supervolt machines produce precisely and carefully calculated high-energy rays, which can be aimed directly at a specific portion of the body—such as the prostate—sparing most of the normal, healthy tissue nearby. Another way of administering radiation is through internal radiation; this involves placing radioactive material directly into the body.

If the urologist recommends that a patient undergo radiotherapy for prostate cancer, he will refer the patient to a physician known as a radiotherapist or radiation oncologist. This specialist will plan and supervise the radiation treatment. Treatments are usually given (on an out-patient basis) over a period of six or seven weeks—usually in a clinic, hospital, or specially equipped office. A machine is aimed at the patient in such a way as to direct the radiation at the specific area selected by the radiotherapist (in collaboration with the urologist). There is no pain or discomfort involved in the procedure, which is much the same as having an ordinary x-ray picture taken. But the results can be dramatic: radiotherapy can result in cure or complete control of prostatic cancer, especially if it is undertaken in the early stages of the disease. The treatment is extended over time so that the doses of radiation can remain small, in order to minimize reactions in the rectum and bladder (both of which lie close to the prostate).

Radiation therapy may also be offered to patients whose cancer has only spread a bit beyond the prostate. In these instances, the radiation is directed toward the whole pelvic area, in order to include all of the pelvic lymph nodes. If the cancer has spread to the bones, radiation may be directed toward the areas affected, to minimize pain and also to help the patient avoid fractures that might otherwise result from even such relatively mild injuries as slipping on wet pavement (since metastasis of cancer from the prostate to the weight-bearing bones can cause them to weaken).

Internal radiation is a much newer technique than external radiation, but it is now an established therapy for certain cancers, and has been used to treat cancer of the prostate for many years. Effective results are often obtained by concentrating the radiation within the prostate itself, thus sparing the surrounding tissues. When using this method, a radiotherapist implants radioactive substances in the prostate, and these emit radiation locally.

In some instances, radioactive wires or needles are inserted directly into the prostate in an operating room; these are completely removed within a few days after they are inserted. Since they extend outside of the body, removing them is simple.

Some radioactive implants can be left permanently in the prostate. Such implants are designed to stop emitting radiation within a specified period (usually only a few days) after implantation. These implants do not cause pain or discomfort; and once their radioactivity ends, the patient's friends and family can come close without fear of contamination. Men with permanent implants in their prostates are able to have sexual intercourse with no risk to their partners.

Just as with external radiation, the amount of internal radiation emitted must be very carefully restricted, to avoid damaging the rectum and the bladder. The proper distribution of radioactive sources is of major importance, as is the calculation of the correct dosage. Many major medical centers can perform the implantation procedure. Internal radiation reduces the number and degree of side effects to the rectum and to the bladder; but since it involves an operation, it is less frequently used than external radiation.

Fatigue is a common side effect of both external and internal radiation. Nonetheless, many men are able to continue working while being treated for prostate cancer. Occasionally the patient experiences some skin reactions in the area toward which external treatment has been directed. This is because the radiation must pass through the skin of the treatment area to reach the cancerous cells in the tissues below. Radiation side effects can be minimized by avoiding use of strong or perfumed soaps, colognes, heat lamps, and hotwater bottles. If skin does become red, flaky, or itchy, plain cornstarch can be used as a soothing powder.

Radiation sometimes causes nausea, cramps, urinary frequency, vomiting, and diarrhea. The physician can prescribe medication to control these effects. Eating lightly before and after treatment and avoiding hot, spicy foods can help to control these problems, too. Loss of appetite may also occur as a result of radiation therapy, followed by weight loss. Eating tempting, nutritious high-protein snacks whenever hungry and trying to make eating time a pleasant, sociable hour encourages better nutritional intake.

Generally, nurses who work with radiotherapists can offer other suggestions on ways to cope with any radiation side effects.

Patients occasionally wonder why some urologists recommend radical surgery for localized prostate cancer while others recommend radiation therapy. In the past, when given a choice, many patients preferred radiation—either external or internal—to surgery because impotence was less likely to result. However, the risk of impotence did exist with radiation—and still does. According to a number of studies, between 20 and 50 percent of all men who undergo radiation therapy for prostate cancer become impotent. With the new nerve-sparing surgery developed by Dr. Walsh, only about 30 percent of all patients so treated become impotent. These percentages are based on *all* men who undergo the specified procedures; in either case, the younger the man, the less likely he is to be rendered impotent.

Which method is more likely to offer a cure for localized prostatic cancer—radiotherapy or surgery? Unfortunately, there is no definitive answer. Both are considered effective forms of treatment, and studies suggest (but do not yet prove) that the survival rates of patients are the same for both. As yet, however, long-term follow-up studies do not exist to permit a conclusion about the ability of radiation therapy to be as effective as surgery. For this reason, many urologists feel that surgical therapy offers a more clearcut opportunity for disease control than is offered by radiation.

HORMONAL TREATMENTS

Since prostatic cancer depends in almost all instances on male hormones for growth, a bilateral orchiectomy (removal of both testicles) is often recommended for patients whose cancer has spread beyond the prostatic capsule. Men who prefer not to have this surgery done opt to achieve the same result by taking estrogen, a female hormone. Estrogen is administered in the form of small pills, taken on a regular basis. Generally, the recommended dosage is 3 milligrams of diethylstilbestrol (DES) per day. Some years ago, doctors noticed that cardiac conditions arose in many patients who were taking larger doses of the drug. The risk of this effect is reduced considerably, however, by giving the patient much smaller amounts, and studies show that these lower doses are equally effective as larger doses in slowing the growth of cancer and in reversing some of the symptoms that appear if the cancer has spread to the bones.

In many men, estrogens reduce libido and limit the ability to achieve an erection. Even in small doses, the female hormone can cause some enlargement of a man's breasts (gynecomastia). To avoid this side effect—which occurs in a small proportion of men—a patient may ask to receive small doses of radiation beforehand in each breast, preventing growth of the breasts while they are under hormonal influence.

DES may cause some lessening of beard and some alteration of body shape. Men who previously were very thin and athletic-looking may become fatter and thinner-skinned. Generally, these changes are hardly noticeable to anyone but the patient himself, and they can be minimized if he stays in good shape through proper diet and exercise.

These feminizing effects occur because the female hormones cause the testes to atrophy (shrink), thereby reducing the quantity of androgens (male hormones) in the body. The results resemble those achieved by removal of the testicles.

Leuprolide is a fairly new drug that is offered to patients whose cancer has spread beyond the prostatic capsule. This drug is administered by means of injection. Leuprolide suppresses the male hormones and seems to have as good a therapeutic effect as DES. Its side effects are similar to those of DES. Other hormones and antiandrogens are also used; a once-a-month injection of a drug related to Leuprolide, called Zolodex, is now being widely studied.

Some premature media publicity followed the announcement of a study being conducted by Ferdinand Labrie, M.D., at Laval University in Quebec, in which two different drugs were being used to treat men with advanced prostate cancer. Initial results of tests were encouraging, and many people jumped to the conclusion that a cure had been found for such cancers, but a great deal of additional research is needed before the study attains scientific validity.

Sometimes hormonal treatment is used for patients with a localized incidence of cancer. According to a leading endocrinologist, J. Lester Gabrilove, M.D. (Professor of Medicine at the Mount Sinai School of Medicine), who has conducted a number of studies of Leuprolide in collaboration with Michael Droller, M.D. (chairman of the Department of Urology in the same institution), this treatment is suitable for various patients who are not good candidates for surgery—men who have other illnesses that put them at high risk for surgery, men who are fearful of surgery and do not mind becoming impotent, and elderly men who might benefit from small doses of medication as a prevention against the spread of the cancer.

CHEMOTHERAPY

Chemotherapy is the treatment of cancer (or any other disease) by means of a combination of different chemical substances or drugs that work internally and invisibly throughout the body. Chemotherapy actually kills cancer cells. Hormones are often viewed as being an adjunct of chemotherapy because they are often used prior to or concurrently with chemotherapy.

Dr. Ezra M. Greenspan, Clinical Professor of Medicine (oncology) at the Mount Sinai School of Medicine, and medical director of the Chemotherapy Foundation, Inc., remains optimistic about the potential effectiveness of combination chemotherapy as a treatment for cancer of the prostate. He explains that new drugs are constantly being developed that are effective against various cancers, and he notes that the use of the individual agents, singly and in combination with each other and with hormones, is constantly being evaluated as a means for treating prostate cancer. Although chemotherapy is not among the primary treatment methods for cancer of the prostate, it is an essential component of the treatment plan for some patients—especially those who have responded poorly to hormone therapy alone. Certain groups of patients have shown increased rates of survival and improved levels of relief from symptoms and pain as a result of receiving chemotherapy.

Many urologists are reluctant to recommend chemotherapy because not all specialists agree that it is effective, and because it has some unpleasant side effects, including nausea, hair loss, chronic fatigue, and a general feeling of illness. To some extent, these effects can be lessened; the patient's physician or the nurse may suggest some ways to accomplish this.

IMMUNOTHERAPY AND OTHER NEW TREATMENTS

Immunotherapy—the attempt to stimulate and strengthen the body's own natural defenses against disease—is still fairly new and is being used in combination with chemotherapy to treat advanced prostate cancer. When used with chemotherapy, it is sometimes referred to as *chemoimmunotherapy*. Among the forms of immunotherapy that have been developed are BCG (bacillus Calmette-Guerin), which is a mixture of live organisms, and Interferon, which is named after its ability to interfere with virus infections. Both have been demonstrated to be effective against some cancers. As yet, neither substance has been shown to be effective against prostate cancer, but studies continue.

PALLIATIVE THERAPY

Palliation is treatment that is not aimed at curing the patient, but at making him feel better by relieving symptoms, pain, or discomfort caused by a disease.

For example, a urologist may perform a TUR on a

patient who has prostate cancer; the purpose in this case is not to treat the cancer, but to deal with urinary blockage that has resulted from the cancer or from BPH coexisting with the cancer. This treatment can afford the patient comfort and can prevent complications such as kidney failure. Urologists usually postpone such measures until after cancer treatment has begun, however, because the cancer treatment may sometimes help relieve the obstruction.

If prostate cancer has spread to the patient's bones, pain may result. While the degree of pain felt may not be related to the severity of the disease (as shown by a bone scan), it can and should be treated.

Aspirin and other antiinflammatory drugs are often sufficient palliatives, but if pain is more severe, stronger drugs can be offered. Many nonnarcotic pain relievers work well; if they do not in a particular case, narcotics can be used. Drugs can be taken in tablet, capsule, or liquid form, or they can be delivered by means of a pump that is either implanted or worn next to the body. Many men take pride in their ability to withstand pain, so they are reluctant to use strong drugs; others are fearful of becoming addicted to such drugs, knowing that drug addicts commonly develop behavioral changes, a craving for the drug, and personality disorders. According to physicians who specialize in pain management, however, this rarely occurs in cancer patients; less than 1 percent of all cancer patients treated for pain are at risk of becoming addicted to the drugs used for this purpose.

Despite knowing this, many physicians and family members hesitate to give cancer patients sufficient medication to relieve their pain—and when such help is offered, some patients foolishly refuse it.

Sometimes, if pain is severe but limited to a single area

(such as the hips or the pelvic region), local radiation can provide prompt, long-lasting, and effective pain relief.

In some instances, a nerve block is administered. This is a procedure in which a substance such as alcohol, cortisone, phenol, or an anesthetic is injected into or around a nerve, providing temporary or permanent relief. It is even possible to cut or destroy nerves, thereby permanently eliminating feeling (and hence pain) in the affected area.

Two other approaches to pain relief are only occasionally used. Hypophysectomy (removal of the pituitary gland) and adrenalectomy (removal of the adrenal glands) reduce the production of male hormones and pain to the bones. At one time removal of the pituitary gland required surgery through the skull, but today the surgical route proceeds through the upper gum and the nasal passage, and from there into the pituitary, which is located below the brain.

Other, nonmedical approaches to pain relief can be very helpful to the patient. Biofeedback, which helps the patient recognize, modify, and control certain involuntary habits or bodily responses, can relax and improve the condition of cancer patients who suffer from anxiety, tension, and muscle pain as a reaction to the disease and its treatment.

Skin stimulation involves the use of pressure, heat, cold, vibration, electrical stimulation, or menthol preparations. All of these have a role in the management of pain. Electrical stimulation transmitted to nerves through a procedure called *transcutaneous electric nerve stimulation* (TENS) is especially effective in treating localized pain. The patient wears a small battery-powered pack or box that is no larger than a cigarette pack. Electrodes from the box are placed on the skin at various trigger points. When pain is felt, the patient simply switches on the mild electrical current, which temporarily blocks the pain—often providing hours of relief. The patient's personal physician, perhaps in conjunction with a physical therapist, can offer advice on how to obtain and operate a TENS device.

Diversion, imagery, meditation, and relaxation can help take the patient's mind off pain and thus relieve pain. Some psychotherapists specialize in helping patients learn these techniques.

Pain is not an unavoidable part of prostate cancer—even if the cancer has spread to the bones. The patient's urologist or personal physician, or the pain management specialist at his local hospital should be able to help identify the means necessary to achieve this relief.

UNPROVED AND DANGEROUS METHODS

Newly approved drugs, when administered with the careful supervision of doctors using established medical guidelines, are worth considering—even though they may not yet have an extensive record of effectiveness. But every few years, an unproved cancer treatment is introduced and becomes available to the public. Many of these are not only ineffective, but downright harmful. A few years ago, for example, the drug Laetrile appeared on the market. It was cyanide-laden and toxic, and the National Cancer Institute determined that it was useless. In addition to various worthless "wonder drugs," an unending supply of vitamins, fad diets (including the macrobiotic diet), "immunoaugmentative therapy" (a treatment derived from various parts of human blood), and other so-called "cures" is pedaled to the public. Usually, detailed case histories of their effects are not published in reliable medical journals, nor is the medical community offered reports of the initial results of treatment, as it is by researchers conducting established studies. Although many of these treatments do no actual harm by themselves, some *are* harmful; and believers often rely on them so heavily that they forgo medically established treatment. Too many people waste precious time and savings on scientifically suspect drugs when more reliable treatments are available. At this time, *no* diet has been proved to cure prostatic cancer or any other kind of cancer, despite claims to the contrary. A patient who hears about some new treatment but has any doubts about its efficacy, should contact the American Cancer Society. It maintains an updated list of materials on unproved methods of cancer management, which is available from its national office. Anyone who has questions about *any* cancer treatment should call the ACS or the National Cancer Institute, whose Cancer Information Service (CIS) can be reached at 1-800-4-CANCER.

The assertion (sometimes made) that the medical profession and government agencies are not really interested in finding a cure for cancer is groundless. No doctor or government official is immune to cancer, and most have, at some time, had cancer strike someone close to them. Doctors, like everyone else, hope to see cancer eradicated some day and are constantly reminding patients of the importance of early detection and treatment.

Early diagnosis and early treatment of cancer of the prostate continue to be crucial. Meanwhile, the outlook for control of the disease is improving: of the approximately 96,000 American men who will develop prostatic cancer during the next year, many will live to a ripe old age.

8

ZINC, VITAMINS, AND NUTRITION: EFFECTS ON THE PROSTATE

Patients often ask urologists if it would be helpful for them to take zinc pills, either to prevent prostate problems or to aid in their treatment. There is much controversy about the use of zinc as a means of prevention or therapy for prostatic disease, so it is important to examine both sides of the question.

Zinc is a trace element found in all human beings. It is needed by the human organism in extremely small amounts. According to Victor Herbert, M.D., J.D., professor of medicine at the Mount Sinai School of Medicine in New York and chairman of the Committee to Strengthen Nutrition, zinc deficiency may be experienced by some vegetarians because their diet may be unbalanced and because the excessive fiber in their diet can draw zinc out of the food and into the stool. This can occur even if the individual's diet otherwise would supply enough zinc.

A deficiency of zinc can lead to major medical problems. It has long been known that the absence of zinc in the diet during childhood and adolescence can cause retardation of physical growth, delayed sexual development, impaired growth of hair, and roughness of skin.

Some evidence indicates that a pregnant woman who is zinc-deficient may have a child who remains at risk for immune deficiency well into the teenage years. Any diet that supplies less than 10 milligrams of zinc per day is likely to cause some serious disturbances in the functioning of the body's organs and glands. Zinc is thought to play an essential role in the immune response of adults as well as of children, and some evidence suggests that it may have a positive effect on the common cold. In addition, it is necessary to the sensations of taste buds, disposal of carbon dioxide and maintaining acid levels in the stomach.

Zinc is found in high concentration in seminal fluid and in the prostate gland itself, which contains more zinc than any other organ in the body. The reason for this high level of zinc in the prostate and in its secretions, however, is not known. Studies of zinc and the prostate have been conducted at many research centers, but no conclusive, universally acknowledged evidence has yet shown that taking zinc pills can prevent or clear up a man's prostatic disease.

ZINC-PROSTATE STUDIES

Dr. William Fair, a urologist at Sloan-Kettering Memorial Medical Center in New York, and formerly the chairman of the Division of Urology at Washington University School of Medicine, has for many years been interested in the relationship between zinc and the prostate. He has noted that zinc is important in the prevention of prostatic disease and that it may be important therapeutically as well. The only problem, in his view, is that the prostate fails to pick zinc up when it is taken orally. The zinc clearly gets into the bloodstream, but Dr. Fair concluded that neither the prostatic tissue nor the prostatic fluid draws in the zinc from there. And if the prostate does not receive the zinc, any amelioration or prevention of prostatic disease is unlikely, even if the man persists in taking zinc tablets.

While Dr. Fair was at Washington University Medical School, however, he saw many patients who reported improvement in symptoms of either prostatitis or BPH after taking zinc in foods or in capsule form. But because these patients were also receiving other kinds of treatment, such as prostatic massage, it was difficult to determine which treatment was responsible for the improvement. Dr. Fair agrees with that medical maxim that "whatever a doctor does within good reason and medical responsibility, some patients will get better, some will get worse, and some will remain the same." He also suspects that a placebo effect was at work; that is, if a patient feels that something will make him feel better, it may indeed do that.

In 1988 Dr. Fair reported some additional observations, noting that zinc levels are down in patients with cancer, but adding that "the reason for this is not yet established." He feels that further studies are needed to determine how zinc could get to the prostate. "It needs a carrier," he says, "that is, another substance that will guide the zinc to the prostate, where it can then work to prevent and alleviate symptoms."

Some researchers are focusing on this rather complex relationship between zinc and the prostate because they, like other researchers, have long noted that patients with chronic prostatitis have either a diminished level or a total absence of zinc in their prostatic secretions, as compared to men without prostatic problems. This seems to suggest that the presence of zinc in the prostate may serve as a defense against prostatic and urinary infections. They have definitely found that, in vitro (in a test tube), the amount of zinc normally present in the prostatic fluid is effective against various types of bacteria. Some experts believe that the drop in zinc concentration in prostatic fluid *precedes* any bacterial invasion of the prostate, rather than bacteria causing a drop in the zinc concentration.

But what causes the marked decrease of zinc in the prostatic fluid of patients with chronic prostatitis? And what methods can be used to alter the zinc level in the fluid, as a possible means of eradicating chronic bacterial prostatitis or of increasing the resistance of the patient to the disease? Those questions cannot be answered without further study.

Dr. Irving M. Bush, professor of urology at the Chicago Medical School, and his staff of researchers have been studying zinc and its relation to the prostate for many years. When interviewed in 1988, Dr. Bush said that more and more men are taking zinc, and that it is becoming accepted practice. He feels that zinc is necessary for healthy prostate function; and he himself recommends that patients take zinc sulfate, as do many other urologists. Zinc gluconate, which many people believe helps fight colds, is not effective for the prostate, according to Dr. Bush.

"Zinc plays a role in B-12 metabolism in patients with prostatitis," he says. "In our large study group, we found that oral zinc and B-12 injections have an effect on estradiol [an estrogen] metabolism, which definitely plays a role in prostatitis and *may* play a role in BPH."

Dr. Bush is aware that many researchers believe that the prostate does not get the zinc from the bloodstream when men take zinc supplements. Analyzing the accumulation of zinc in the prostate is a complex undertaking, and Dr. Bush believes that many researchers are not using the proper techniques in their analyses.

Something of a lone ranger among doctors on the zinc question, Dr. Bush says that people are wrong to look for dramatic results: "You can't take it for ten days and feel better. It's a long range thing over a long period. But I note that more and more doctors are using it, and they are finding that patients seemingly do better in the long run with than without it."

Dr. Bush feels that zinc is helpful in patients with congestive prostatitis because their bodies do not have enough available zinc. There are, of course, individual differences in zinc needs. Diabetics, who need zinc in order to utilize insulin, and heavy drinkers, who require zinc in order to break down alcohol in the liver—as well as individuals with other conditions not completely understood at this time—have an increased need for zinc. Some doctors also believe that individuals undergoing unusual stress require additional zinc.

In those instances, the pituitary gland sends a message to the prostate to filter more zinc, and in the prostate's effort to do this, congestion or enlargement of the glands may occur. The situation resembles borrowing from Peter to pay Paul: the zinc needed by other parts of the body is taken from the prostate, and the prostate thereupon becomes zinc-starved. In its efforts to free up more zinc, the prostate gets into trouble.

Dr. Bush explains that this pattern is analagous to the one seen in patients with thyroid conditions. The thyroid gland stores iodine, and if a shortage of iodine occurs in the thyroid, the gland enlarges. If iodine is administered to the patient early enough after enlargement begins, the thyroid shrinks back to its normal size. If medical help is postponed and the thyroid becomes greatly enlarged, the iodine may no longer be able to shrink the thyroid, but it still keeps the gland from continuing to enlarge.

Dr. Bush finds that zinc therapy is effective for BPH if it is begun when the prostate first starts to enlarge. The zinc in the body, he explains, keeps the prostate's glandular tissue from enlarging in order to produce zinc. Although zinc supplements will not shrink the enlarged fibrous and muscular tissue, they *can* shrink the glandular tissue and thus afford the patient much relief. Many patients with BPH also have some form of prostatitis, and the zinc will also help improve this condition. Dr. Bush says that his patients report having a better sense of well-being from the combined zinc and vitamin therapy, and also report urinating more comfortably and making far fewer bathroom trips at night (because the glandular tissue shrinks). Dr. Bush says that he continues to provide prostatic massages but finds that they become less necessary for many of his patients. Most important, he is able to avoid performing surgery on an increasing number of these patients.

OBSERVING ZINC THERAPY

Dr. Bush reminds all of his patients that, although they are feeling much better and are showing fewer symptoms, it is essential that they continue to be monitored carefully. He regularly conducts diagnostic tests of kidney function, and his patients have their semen and blood measured periodically for zinc content. He also does regular semen cultures to check on bacteria.

In earlier studies, Dr. Bush only used zinc therapy on patients for a few months, but he and his researchers now keep patients on zinc therapy for longer periods of time; some have already been on the therapy for twenty years. He says, "These men seem to need prostate surgery at a far lesser rate than other patients." In the past five years, he and his researchers have looked at 5,000 patients, so his view that zinc helps to shrink the prostate is not an expression of pure abstract theory. In his opinion, orally administered zinc definitely gets to the prostate. "No doubt about it," he declares.

Dr. Bush says that the zinc formula he prescribes contains additional vitamins and minerals; he feels that this combination leads to far better results than can be obtained when zinc is used alone. He stresses that, while zinc may ordinarily be used in moderation by a patient (along with regular daily vitamins), no man should try to prescribe zinc for himself to treat prostate problems. A doctor's supervision is essential, and of course every man over forty should have regular rectal examinations. A man who is suffering from any prostatic symptoms should receive thorough urological examinations regularly, whether or not he is using zinc.

Dr. Bush also offers patients a combination of zinc and alpha-2 blockers. He continues rectal massage, as well, which he says is particularly helpful for patients who have enlarged seminal vesicles—a condition that he believes is sometimes mistaken by urologists for an enlarged prostate.

Many urologists who have been asked by patients about zinc have responded by putting them on a regimen of zinc tablets and a diet that includes zinc-rich foods. These patients often report a decrease in symptoms and (equally important) a general sense of well-being. This confirms observations made in the Greenberger office.

An interesting study was conducted at the University of Missouri Medical School involving seventy infertile men with chronic infectious prostatitis who were treated by prostatic massage, drug therapy, and injections of zinc or vitamins directly into the prostate. The results of the study were not conclusive, but they suggest that the addition of the zinc helped in clearing up the bacteria.

ZINC-RICH FOODS

Eating zinc-rich foods may help bolster prostatic health. Foods that are rich in zinc include seafood (especially oysters), nuts, pumpkin seeds, sunflower seeds, wheat bran, wheat germ, brewer's yeast, milk, eggs, onions, molasses, poultry, peas, beans, lentils, meat (especially beef liver), and gelatin. Unfortunately some of these foods (such as eggs and liver) are high in cholesterol or fat or may be bad for a person's general health. Another problem in trying to rely upon diet to obtain zinc is that it is almost nonexistent in refined processed foods. Careless cooking and soil exhaustion have reduced the number of high-zinc sources available to us to considerably less than the preceding list would indicate.

If the soil in which food grows is deficient in zinc (as much of it is), the food will be deficient, too. If the animals from which we obtain the food are deficient in zinc, their products will also be deficient. The best way to obtain natural zinc is to use garden-fresh (not just market-fresh) vegetables and to cook them slowly at a low temperature, or eat them raw. Although oysters are generally rich in zinc, the waters in which they live are often contaminated, diminishing the natural level of zinc, if not altogether destroying it. Moreover, oysters (like liver) are bad for gout. In order for people to obtain their recommended daily allowance of 15 milligrams of zinc, they may have to take zinc supplements. And a man who plans to use zinc as a protective or therapeutic agent against prostatic disease would be well advised to take zinc supplements, rather than to rely on diet.

As in dealing with any vitamin, mineral, or medication, a person must remember the old adage that "too much of a good thing is bad for you," and not take too much zinc. How much is too much? The amount varies from person to person and should be determined in consultation with each individual's personal physician. Most doctors seem to feel that an appropriate therapeutic dose is 50 milligrams daily, and many say that 150 milligrams is the maximum amount a patient can tolerate without adverse side effects. The side effects—which may include diarrhea, nausea, and vomiting—are seldom serious if checked in time, but they can be extremely uncomfortable. One word of caution: some physicians believe that large doses of zinc may diminish the body's level of selenium (another metallic element), which is widely thought to have a protective effect against cancer. In addition to causing these side effects, a very high dose of zinc can inhibit the immune system and lower a person's white blood cell count.

Foods that are rich in zinc have been used for thousands of years to treat various medical ills. Zinc has long been known to be effective in helping to heal wounds; present studies indicate that it also has a definite place in the healing of chronic ulcers, burns, and hepatitis, and that it may have a place in postsurgical healing. Its effect on recovery from prostatic surgery has not yet been established.

Pumpkin seeds, which are generally rich in zinc, have long been believed by many nutritionists and physicians to be effective in aiding prostatic health, as well as sexual and neurological dysfunction. Almost fifty years ago, it was noted that BPH was almost nonexistent in Transylvania. Pumpkin seeds were an important part of the diet of Transylvanians, and it is tempting to conclude that there is some connection between the two.

Some theorists feel that zinc supplements may only be helpful if a deficiency of the element already exists, but this has not been proved either. It is possible, of course, that some men's metabolism of zinc may be such that they require more than others do to maintain prostatic health. In other words, an adequate amount of zinc for one man may be too little for another man, even if he does not have any special condition that would seem to require extra zinc.

VITAMINS IN FOODS AND SUPPLEMENTS

Many nutritionists and physicians consider vitamins A, C, D, and E to be important in maintaining good prostatic health; as a result, they recommend that men take supplementary vitamins (readily available in grocery and drug stores), and encourage them to eat a diet rich in these vitamins. Some experts believe that unsaturated fatty acids and pollen tablets may be helpful, too. Foods rich in vitamin A include calf and beef liver, chicken liver, spinach, turnip greens, cabbage, string beans, broccoli, carrots, yellow squash, apricots, sweet potatoes, and yams. The presence of vitamin E is necessary to prevent destruction of vitamin A, so the diet must also include plenty of vitamin E. The U.S. Recommended Daily Allowance of vitamin A for most adults is 5,000 international units (I.U.), and anywhere from 10,000 to 20,000 I.U. per day can usually be consumed without causing any problems. Too much vitamin A can be toxic, so a greater-than-normal supplement of the vitamin should not be taken without close medical supervision.

Orange juice is the best known supplier of vitamin C, but broccoli, green peppers, brussels sprouts, strawberries, and cabbage also provide it—and with fewer calories. All citrus fruits and tomatoes are good sources of vitamin C. The U.S. RDA is 60 milligrams, but therapeutic doses range from 200 to 500 milligrams, and some nutritionists recommend even more. Excesses should be avoided because they pose a risk of forming kidney stones. Magnesium supplements should be taken along with large doses of Vitamin C, to help prevent this problem.

Vitamin D is found in vitamin D–enriched milk, in fish liver oils, in salmon, in tuna, in sardines, in egg yolks, and in margarine. The U.S. RDA is 400 I.U., and self-therapy should not include more than about 1,000 I.U. daily, since serious toxic effects can result from too much vitamin D.

Vitamin E is found in wheat germ, whole grain bread, rice, safflower oil, vegetable oils, peanuts, and green leafy vegetables such as cabbage, spinach, asparagus, and broccoli. The U.S. RDA for adults is 30 I.U. per day, and supplements should range from 30 to 100 I.U. Some nutritionists recommend taking up to 600 I.U. per day, but since persons with high blood pressure, diabetes, or rheumatic heart conditions should take only the minimum supplements, it is highly advisable to discuss the matter with a physician before embarking on a regimen of vitamin E beyond the range of 30 to 60 I.U. per day.

Fatty acids are also widely considered to be important to prostatic health. Polyunsaturated fatty acids are found in vegetable oils and fish oils, and they do not raise the body's cholesterol level. Essential fatty acid capsules (up to 1,200 milligrams per day) may be of therapeutic value in reducing the size of an enlarged prostate. Other good food sources of fatty acids are unrefined seeds, whole grains, and cold-pressed vegetable oils such as soybean oil, safflower oil, sunflower oil, and corn oil.

Lecithin, a substance found in egg yolks, is also considered important to prostatic health. Daily supplements of 1 to 2 tablespoons, in granular, powder, or liquid form, may be helpful.

Some studies in Sweden and Japan indicate that a pollen preparation called *cernitin* is very useful in treating prostatitis. Pollen tablets are available at drug and health food stores; a recommended therapeutic dose is three tablets daily.

What a man does not eat may be even more important than what he does eat, as far as prostatic health is concerned. Spicy foods, coffee, and alcohol irritate the prostate and should be avoided by men who already have prostatic problems. Men interested in prevention should consume these products in moderation. Zinc supplements may be extremely helpful to a man who drinks more beer, wine, or spirits than he should because zinc can be helpful in breaking down alcohol in the liver. An even wiser step would be to cut down on or eliminate consumption of alcohol.

Generally speaking, the rules of good nutrition apply to everyone: man, woman, or child. Further information on this topic can be obtained from some of the books listed at the back of this book.

To a man who is reaching the age at which prostatic problems are most likely to arise, good diet is essential. Following some of the suggestions given in this chapter may be an extremely helpful way to begin improving a diet. Although much of the value of zinc, vitamins, and other supplements to prostatic health remains in the exploratory stage, and although the statistics are not conclusive, use of such supplements is certainly worth considering. But—and this is important in all strategies of self-care—a person should never rely exclusively on diet, vitamins, or minerals for good health. Everyone should see his personal physician regularly, even if he is feeling well. Before beginning on any new diet or regimen of vitamins, he should discuss it with the doctor. A particular diet or vitamin dose may be extremely unwise for someone who has any other medical problem or condition. It is best that the doctor know what the patient is taking and that the doctor keep a record of it in the patient's chart. Then, if any new symptoms arise, the doctor can investigate the possibility of its being an allergic or toxic reaction to a vitamin or a new food—even if the dose taken is within the range of a usual therapeutic dose.

9

SOCIAL AND SEXUAL ACTIVITY AFTER PROSTATE SURGERY

One evening in the late 1970s, 500 retired people attended a talk at which various health professionals (including Dr. Greenberger and the author) discussed issues of great importance to them. The audience enjoyed Dr. Greenberger's opening remarks on the subject of prostate problems and sexual activities in the later years:

Many years ago, when I was a young urologist, an elderly patient was referred to me as a candidate for prostate surgery. He was miserable because of urinary blockage, but the man refused to consent to surgery until he fully discussed with me the effects the operation might have on his sexual activity. I had already taken a full medical, social, and sexual history from him, and I knew that this man had not engaged in sexual activity for many years. I wondered aloud why he was so concerned. He pointed out of the window at the Statue of Liberty and said, "See her over there? I haven't visited her in more than twenty years, but I do like knowing she's there."

His point was well made, and I never forgot it. I realized then that every man likes to know "it"—the ability to function sexually, when and if he wants to—"is still there."

118

Virtually any man who is contemplating prostatic surgery worries about how the operation will affect his social life and—especially—his sex life. This is true regardless of whether the man has been sexually active or not, and regardless of whether he has a regular partner or is simply on the lookout for Ms. Right.

Consequently, most urologists fully inform their patients concerning the possible effects of an impending prostatectomy on their sexual ability. Sometimes the patient's wife is the one who asks first about how the prostatectomy will affect the man's sexual performance. In essence, the answer on that point is always the same: for the most part, if the man was able to have an erection and engage in sex prior to surgery, he will be able to do so after surgery. If he could not or did not before, the situation is not likely to change after surgery—at least not without special counseling or treatment.

The experiences of the Greenberger associates have been borne out in several studies done throughout the country. The type of surgery—whether TUR, suprapubic prostatectomy or retropubic prostatectomy—usually does not affect erectile functioning. For greater than 80 percent of men, sexual functioning returns to the presurgical level; about 10 percent improve; and about 10 percent lose some ability. Generally, the men who lose some or all sexual ability are in the oldest age group (over seventy), and most were only occasionally active prior to surgery.

When a change in sexual activity does accompany prostate problems or surgery for BPH, it is usually not related either to the original condition or to the surgery itself. Instead, it is related to the age of the man, the way he views himself, and his life in general.

119

URINARY INCONTINENCE

Sometimes (but not usually), a man may have a problem controlling the flow of urine from his body following prostate surgery due to sphincter muscle damage. This is quite rare after surgery for BPH but a bit more common after surgery for cancer—although less so since the development of the new nerve-sparing surgery. Although urinary incontinence in itself does not cause impotence, it *can* embarrass the man and lower his sense of self-esteem, which can discourage him from even attempting intimacy. Moreover, concern over incontinence can lead a man to restrict his social activities to a minimum, profoundly altering his life-style and severely limiting the ways in which he can enjoy himself from day to day.

If incontinence occurs, the patient should consult his urologist, who will carefully investigate the causes to determine the best method of treatment. The urologist will conduct tests called *urodynamics*—x-ray studies that help gauge how well the patient's bladder and urinary sphincter muscle are functioning—and he may also cystoscope the patient.

An irritative (uninhibited) bladder may respond well to antispasmodic medications. Overflow incontinence (continuous distention of bladder with dribbling of urine) can have a neurological cause, or it may signal that the prostate is still obstructing the urethra; if the latter condition exists, additional corrective surgery may be indicated.

If surgery or radiation has damaged the urinary sphincter muscle, treatment with medication may be successful. Alternatively, it is possible to have an artificial sphincter implanted in the body through an incision in the lower abdomen and (sometimes) behind the scrotum. Squeezing a pump opens the urethra, enabling the patient to urinate; after urination, the device automatically closes. Urologists can provide further information on this device.

Exercises and biofeedback have been very successful in reversing incontinence in some people; most urologists can refer patients to a specialist in these methods. If the incontinence cannot be reversed, other ways of coping with the problem can be pursued.

Some people may choose to wear absorbent, disposable undergarments, others may use a drip collector, which is a cuplike or pouchlike device that collects small amounts of urine.

Internal collection devices similar to the catheters used after surgery can be left in place, draining into a leg bag. The catheter will be replaced by the urologist from time to time. The bag, which requires frequent emptying, can be worn under regular clothes without being detectable. Unfortunately, it may be necessary for the patient to remain on antibiotics for the duration because of an increased risk of urinary tract infections from the continued insertion of the catheter and from urine remaining in the bladder.

Some men are able to catheterize themselves intermittently, inserting a catheter into their own urethra every few hours (lubricating first). By this means, they are able to empty their bladders completely.

Some men find that a condomlike device that fits over the penis and drains urine into a tube constitutes an effective means of coping with incontinence. Others find it difficult to keep the collection tube in place—even by means of a belt, leg bands, or adhesive.

In any case, incontinence need not lead to a depreciation in self-esteem, nor to a curtailment of activities that the man takes pleasure in—including sexual activity.

EXPERIENCING SEXUALITY IN LATER YEARS

Sexual experiences, like other experiences, are perceived differently by different people—in part because of their individual personalities, but also because of differences in their age. An analogy can be drawn to trimming a Christmas tree or preparing the house for Passover, which likewise gives people of all ages pleasure. The youngest usually focus on the doing and accomplishing. Middle-aged people tune in more to the sense of the holidays as well as the activity. The oldest take their time about it, using an extra hour or so in trimming a tree, an extra day or so in preparing a house properly for Passover. But the overall process is no more tiring, no less satisfying, and in many ways much more pleasurable for them.

This pleasure can be felt in many of the activities and experiences of the later years, including sex. But too often people in their sixties and seventies decide that it is time for sexual relations to stop. If their sexual relationships were never good, they use advancing age as an excuse; and for some of them, this may be an appropriate answer—a sad answer, but perhaps the right one if neither partner feels deprived. But for individuals who once took pleasure in loving and sex, age (in the absence of illness) is no reason to stop. Neither is prostatic surgery a reason to stop.

Older people have the capacity to function sexually and to enjoy it, but they need to know what physiological changes to expect with aging. Then they can not only compensate for these changes, but also turn them to their advantage. A general slowdown in sexual arousal and response are two of the most noticeable changes. All too often, a couple misunderstands these signs. The husband thinks his ability to make love is almost gone, and his wife thinks she must have lost her allure. They wonder why the man takes so long to get ready. When he does perform, why does he sometimes not ejaculate? And when he does ejaculate, why does he lose his erection so rapidly? All of these occurrences are normal; the couple just does not know it.

The man figures that maybe something is wrong—but not with his wife: she still looks great. So he asks his personal physician to check him out. Since he feels no pain, and has experienced no urinary problems, he sees no need to go to a urologist. His personal physician, who may be a nice young fellow, says to his patient, "Well, Jim, you are sixty-five. That happens." And Jim, who came in search of some sensible advice and reassurance that he is sexually okay, leaves with the feeling that he's on the verge of impotence.

Often men who have had this type of experience eventually come to a urologist's office for some other reason. For example, they might have BPH, totally unrelated to their recent sexual problems. The urologist's office consultation room is a good place to discuss their concerns.

Many men are not aware that advancing age causes a definite slowdown in both the time it takes for sexual arousal and the time needed for ejaculation. A man may need more reassurance from his partner, as well as more tactile stimulation. The period of time it takes for him to achieve another erection (called the *refractory period*) is also longer than it once was. At one time he might have been able to have a number of orgasms in one night; but by age sixty, he may need a refractory period of from twenty-four to forty-eight hours between erections. An older man's erection is likely to be less firm than a younger man's and collapses almost immediately after ejaculation. There may be less force to his ejaculation.

Of course, if a man is not prepared for these natural changes, he and his wife may become anxious.

For a man, *fear* of poor performance can *cause* poor performance and is, in fact, the most frequent cause of psychological impotence. Men who understand that these physiological changes are normal and need not affect the quality (or even quantity) of their sexual encounters can relax and continue to enjoy their sexuality as it is.

Another change that accompanies the aging process is the diminished urgency to ejaculate at the climax of every sexual experience. The experience is nonetheless satisfying and fulfilling. Many men are surprised to discover that it is possible to have an orgasm without ejaculation; that is, they can sometimes have the contractions of orgasm—and the satisfying pleasure that it brings—without having any emission of semen.

RETROGRADE EJACULATION

Retrograde ejaculation occurs when the semen goes back into the bladder, rather than through the urethra and out of the penis. Ordinarily the bladder neck closes and the sphincter in the urogenital diaphragm opens at the time of orgasm, so that the sperm is driven down and out of the urethra and penis by the contracting muscles of the urethra. But after surgery, when the channel has been sufficiently widened to allow the urine to flow, the bladder neck may be left permanently open, causing the contractions of the muscles of the urethra to drive the semen upward through the open internal sphincter and into the bladder. The fluid is then expelled the next time a man urinates. Another consequence of this surgery is that the available quantity of ejaculatory fluid will be diminished anyway because one of its sources (the prostate gland) has been partially or completely removed.

Sometimes a man is not initially aware that retrograde ejaculation is happening until his partner calls his attention to it. She may think that he no longer "enjoys" sex, since he does not ejaculate; and he may wonder if she is right, despite the pleasure he has experienced. Prior to a TUR, a suprapubic prostatectomy, or a retropubic prostatectomy, the urologist will explain that retrograde ejaculation will probably result.

While retrograde ejaculation does not affect the sensation of orgasm, nor diminish its pleasure, it usually does mean that the man is described as sterile. Sometimes men confuse fertility with potency, but these are two distinct things. A man incapable of achieving an erection is termed *impotent,* whether or not his body can produce sperm. A man incapable of producing sperm, is termed *sterile,* whether or not he can achieve an erection.

Although a man is likely to have retrograde ejaculation after surgery for BPH, he and his partner (if she is still of childbearing age) should not depend on retrograde ejaculation as a foolproof method of contraception. It is wise for the man to have his ejaculate from the bladder examined by the urologist to determine whether he is still potentially fertile.

If the man's partner wishes to become pregnant, sperm can be extracted from his urine after retrograde ejaculation and then deposited in the woman's vagina by the method called *artificial insemination.* This is done in a physician's office. A child conceived in this manner is the biological child of both partners.

ERECTIONS AND IMPOTENCE

Messages from the brain cause blood to fill the corpora cavernosa (the two spongy columns in the shaft of the penis), making the penis firm. The columns contain seven times their normal flow of blood during erection. In addition to brain messages, other factors are involved in erection: nerve impulses, muscle reactions, hormone levels, and flow of blood. Thus, erection can occur spontaneously (as any parent of a small boy is fully aware!), or in response to mental and physical stimuli.

Impotence (sometimes referred to as *sexual dysfunction*) is generally defined as the inability of a man to achieve and maintain an erection firm enough for penetration and intercourse. An estimated 10 million men in the United States are affected by this problem. A man who is unable to achieve or maintain an erection can still experience orgasm and be able to ejaculate, because these functions are controlled by different nerves. Moreover, desire may remain the same, regardless of the man's ability to perform sexual intercourse.

The term *impotence* covers a range of situations. Some men are never able to have an erection; others find that they can obtain an erection but are unable to maintain it; and some find that they are only occasionally beset with the problem.

Impotence can be the result of physical causes—usually when blood vessels or nerves are damaged or destroyed, or when the body's balance of hormones is changed. Psychological impotence can have a number of causes, and counseling can often help. At one time most cases of impotence were thought to have psychological causes, but it is now believed that about half of all cases of chronic impotence result from physical problems.

126

PHYSICAL CAUSES OF SEXUAL DYSFUNCTION

The urologist's reassurance to patients about resuming regular sexual activity after prostate surgery helps to eliminate most patients' concerns. But some people have problems anyway—often problems that predate surgery. A careful history can sometimes reveal the reason. To determine whether a man's impotence is based on physiological or psychological reasons, the urologist may ask him a number of questions about his medical and social history, followed by one important question: does the patient ever have an erection—in the morning, during the night, or with masturbation? If the answer is yes, there is probably no physiological reason for the problem.

For as yet unknown reasons, all men who are physically capable of having an erection experience them during sleep, but some people, naturally, have no way of knowing if this occurs to them. A simple way to determine this is to stick a little roll of stamps around the penis. If, in the morning each stamp is torn on the perforations it suggests that the man had an erection. More sophisticated tests are also available. One of these makes use of a small fabric band to which plastic strips are attached. It is usually suggested that a man wear this for two consecutive nights. If all of the plastic strips break during the man's sleep, this result suggests that he can achieve erection. If they do not break, the result strongly suggests that the cause of the man's impotence is physical. Many urologists now send patients to a specialist or to a treatment center with expertise in the area of sexual dysfunction for further testing and/or treatment.

Sleep studies can also be conducted to measure nocturnal penile tumescence (NPT). If these studies suggest that a man is not having nighttime erections, the physician will probably recommend that he have thorough neurological, endocrinological, and vascular examinations done, which may identify a physical cause for his impotence.

Until all physical explanations for impotence are ruled out, a man should never assume that his impotence is psychological. But there are many psychological explanations for why a man who was once sexually active may become unable to achieve an erection sufficient for penetration.

After cancer surgery, fear that sexual activity will worsen the cancer or spread it to a partner is quite common, although completely groundless. Anxiety about performance is another frequent cause. A man who is worried about how well he will do and what his partner will think is already in trouble. If he is worried about his partner's receptivity, he may also have problems. The importance of regular sexual activity for older men is a good means of avoiding impotence. "Use it or lose it," many experts say. On the other hand, most urologists have had patients who were sexually inactive for some time because of illness or lack of a partner, but who were able to resume activity when they recovered or found a new partner. Thus, while no urologist would recommend abstinence as a way of preserving sexual ability, sexual inactivity is not necessarily a permanent condition.

Some physical causes of impotence are reversible. In arteriosclerosis, the arteries are clogged and can block blood from passing through the blood vessels leading to the penis. Sometimes, lowering cholesterol levels can help reverse this condition. Smoking, because of its effects on the circulatory system, can be another culprit. Diabetes (or a thyroid condition accompanying it) is the most common cause of impotence; about 2 million men suffer from diabetes-related impotence, which is thought to be related to damage diabetes does to the neural pathways that send messages from spinal cord centers to the penis for erection. Such impotence is often unrelated to whether or not the diabetes is under control, and it can even predate the diagnosis of diabetes. In some instances, tricyclic antidepressants have helped to reverse nerve damage in diabetes.

Sometimes a diabetic man may have a few experiences in which he fails to achieve an erection, then assumes that this was due to the diabetes, and gives up. It is important for men not to let such occasional experiences undermine their confidence so that they actually become impotent.

Various medications can either reduce desire or cause impotence among older men. Many drugs used for hypertension can cause difficulty with erections, but their effects tend to vary from one individual to another. If a patient is affected adversely, the doctor can often prescribe a different drug that controls high blood pressure just as well, without having an unwelcome effect upon sexual ability. Digitalis, which is used for heart failure, can also cause sexual dysfunction.

Some of the drugs used in treating depression tend to interfere with libido and sexual functioning, even though they act as a stimulant for other activities. It should be noted, however, that depressed individuals often have sexual problems already. Sedatives, tranquilizers, chemotherapy, cold medications, and even eyedrops used for glaucoma can cause performance problems, as well.

Alcohol consumption commonly has a deleterious effect on sexual function. Chronic alcoholism can cause impotence in a man of any age, but even a few drinks too many can temporarily cause it in older men. Marijuana and anabolic steroid abuse can also lead to impotence.

Zinc deficiencies, which are common in kidney dialysis patients, can result in impotence. When the lost zinc is replaced, however, the impotence is often reversed.

COUNSELING AND OTHER MEANS OF COPING

If a thorough medical and urological checkup performed by a physician who has special expertise in the area of sexual function rules out physical reasons for impotence, counseling can be extremely helpful.

Many couples benefit from the reassurance about physiological soundness that a urologist can provide, and they may never need to seek further help. Many people simply need to understand more about the sexual changes that occur as they reach their middle (and later) years. The sexual slowdown many men experience can be handled in much the same spirit as traveling to Europe on an ocean liner. An adaptable couple can discover the truth of the slogan, "Getting there is half the fun."

One patient realized this. His wife wrote a letter that remained in the Greenberger files for many years. It was probably written partly in fun.

Dear Dr. Greenberger:
Ever since you operated on my husband, it takes him almost a half hour of lovemaking to achieve an erection, and it's another ten minutes to orgasm. Before his surgery, it took him only five minutes of lovemaking to achieve an erection, and about one minute to have an orgasm. My sister wants to know if you can give her husband the same operation.

Of course, it was not the surgery that made the difference; it was simply the aging process that accompanied the man's BPH, bolstered by the benefits he derived from the frank doctor-patient discussions he had prior to and after surgery.

Other couples have learned that sexual activity is not necessarily synonymous with sexual intercourse. It involves, rather, a much broader realm of human sexuality. Holding, touching, a mutual physical reaching out is just as sexual as genital penetration; and it can be just as satisfying. When people rid themselves of the idea that sexual activity that does not end with intercourse and orgasm is abnormal, they can fully realize their potential as sexual human beings.

When patients do not respond to the information or reassurances of their physician, they should consider referral to a trained and experienced counselor. At the talk in the late 1970s, I described one such case in some detail.

One couple I counseled stands out in my mind. I met him first. He was a lawyer, still in active practice— handsome, grey-haired, age sixty-eight. He had a mischievous grin, but his eyes were sad. As he told me about himself, I could see that he was intelligent and highly creative. His wife, an attractive woman, had been a teacher. Together they had brought up two daughters: one a journalist, the other a lawyer like her father.

For the last seven years this couple had had no sexual contact. None at all. He told it to me this way:

"About seven years ago, I had a prostate operation. Before that our sex life had been just so-so. Sex was just a once-in-a-while thing. After my operation, I felt better than ever. The doctor assured me surgery wouldn't affect my sexual ability. However, the first time we tried, I just couldn't get an erection. The second time was the same. And the third time. I haven't tried since."

"How do you feel about this?" I asked.

"It's not so much the sex act that I miss," he answered. "I miss the touching, the holding, the physical contact. I miss it very much."

In the course of our interviews, I obtained a full history of this couple, and I was able to put together the whole picture.

At one time, they had had a happy and satisfying sex life. But it was mostly focused on performance. He found his wife exciting and took great pride in the fact that he could always get ready quickly. She was flattered and happy that she could elicit this response in him, and much of the time she responded to their lovemaking with enthusiasm, if not always with orgasm. There were times when she didn't much feel like having sex, but she remembered her mother's wedding advice: "If *you* don't, there's always some other woman who will."

So their sex life, never really as full as it might have been, had deteriorated to the point of nonexistence. The husband admitted that it was not only that he missed their old relationship, but that he also wanted what they had never really had. His wife, in separate interviews with me, said much the same thing.

Their lack of communication and the husband's fear of performance had driven them apart sexually, although they still had much in common and shared many good times together. As our session continued and the channels of communication opened up, both were able to speak freely about the lack of their current sex life and what they wanted it to be. The husband confessed that he was afraid if he aroused his wife and then couldn't perform, she would be frustrated and angry. When his wife heard this, she reminded him that penetration is possible even without a full erection, and she said that she could also reach orgasm if he carressed her sexually sensitive areas. Thus, she opened the door for her husband to just enjoy the sensual experience of lovemaking and relieved him of any demand to "perform," so that he did not have to worry about success or failure.

Cases like the preceding one are more common than many people realize. Although fear of failure can lead to sexual dysfunction in both men and women, it is particularly likely to affect men in this way, since women can perform sexually without arousal, but men cannot. This couple's problem was far more closely related to communication than to physiological problems. In any such situation, a man suffering from impotence deserves a full medical workup; then, regardless of the cause, he and his partner may require the help of a specialist in the treatment of sexual dysfunction.

Midlife Love Life (formerly titled *Love and Sex After 40*), coauthored by Pulitzer Prize winner Robert N. Butler, M.D., former director of the National Institute on Aging and now chairman of the Department of Geriatrics and Adult Development of Mount Sinai Medical Center in New York, and Myrna I. Lewis, M.S.W., A.C.S.W., also on the faculty of Mount Sinai, reflects the wisdom and sensitivity of these two clinicians. They describe the normal changes that occur in men and in women during their middle and later years, and they help the reader differentiate among the different causes of sexual dysfunction. They also offer many valuable suggestions about how to cope with changes that occur during the middle and later years.

The new nerve-sparing surgery for cancer of the prostate (described in chapter 7) means that far fewer men experience true impotence after surgery. But some men still have impaired erections or even impotence, either because they have received radiotherapy—which may result in scarring, trauma, or entrapment of nerves—or because they are taking estrogens, other antiandrogens, or chemotherapy for more advanced prostate cancer. Some men are adversely affected by surgery for BPH, but this is quite rare.

A number of men thus affected respond like the older man who has occasional or even chronic trouble achieving a full erection. Knowing that there must have been many occasions when his wife was not really "in the mood" but took pleasure in his pleasure, he can now do the same for her and find that his lovemaking, manual or oral as well as genital, can give her much pleasure and satisfaction. In turn, it can give him much of the pleasure and satisfaction he experienced in earlier years.

Men who feel that there is no substitute or alternative to achieving an erection firm enough for vaginal penetration also have options, but first a word of warning: Unproved and (usually) ineffective treatments for everything from the common cold to advanced cancer to baldness have always been available to those who seek them. So it is with impotence.

Men eager to try anything may resort to vitamins, minerals, and even so-called "aphrodisiacs" offered in ads or in stores. Most of these products are worthless but harmless; some, however, can increase the number of incidents involving impotence, and others can even be physiologically harmful.

Before seeking any such solution to a problem, a man should speak to his urologist or personal physician, who may refer him to a center that specializes in the treatment of sexual dysfunction. A man or his partner can also contact Impotents Anonymous (IA) or ROMP (Recovery of Male Potency)—organizations that offer information and local referrals to professional consultants, as well as support groups. The American Association of Sex Educators, Counselors and Therapists can also refer a man to certified sex counselor-therapists in his area. The addresses and phone numbers of these organizations, along with other relevant sources, are listed in appendix 4.

DRUGS THAT CAN HELP COMBAT IMPOTENCE

Although the Food and Drug Administration (FDA) has banned most aphrodisiacs from being sold over-the-counter, some are sold anyway. Although these preparations may not be labeled as aphrodisiacs, phrases such as "for lifelong vigor," or "specially for men" on the packaging make the intention clear. Small doses of ginseng, available in most health food stores, are popularly believed to enhance sexual health; scientific research suggests that ginseng is harmless but not necessarily helpful. Zinc is necessary for good prostatic health, and a deficiency of it can lead to impotence. Zinc supplements (except to correct a deficiency) are of dubious value in contributing to greater sexual potency, but it is interesting to note that oysters (which are zinc-rich) have long been thought of as an aphrodisiac.

A derivation from an old folk remedy called *yohimbine* is "one aphrodisiac that may at least partially live up to its reputation," says Robert Butler and Myrna Lewis in their book, *Midlife Love Life*. It has received serious attention from physicians and appears to help to restore sexual desire and function to some men. Taken in pill form, it is thought to dilate blocked blood vessels and to spur release of norepinephrine—a compound that is helpful in causing erections. Scientific experimentation with yohimbine continues.

Some urologists recommend injecting a drug called *papaverine* directly into the penis—often in combination with phentolamine mesylate. These medications dilate the arteries in the penis, increasing the flow of blood to the penis, and at the same time dilate the veins so that less blood leaves the penis. This helps an otherwise impotent man achieve and maintain an erection.

135

Papaverine shots have both diagnostic and therapeutic purposes. They can be used to determine if an erection is possible, and they can also be used as a treatment for the condition.

Urologists who recommend this treatment to patients teach the man how to give himself the injections. Using a very small, skinny needle, the man learns to inject the drug into the side of his penis. The needle itself is not painful but the medication causes a mild, very temporary burning sensation. Initially, the man will have injections at the doctor's office to determine his required dose and to make sure he tolerates it well. Occasionally the reactions last for up to a few hours—a situation that may raise the need for immediate medical attention to drain the medication from the penis. Side effects are usually minimal, but they can include nausea and dizziness. A long-term side effect of the treatment is scarring of the penis.

Prostaglandins, naturally occurring hormonelike unsaturated fatty acids, can also serve as vein-dilating agents; they work in much the same way as papaverine does. In some newer experimental studies, prostaglandins are being injected directly into the penis.

Testosterone (a hormone) is sometimes given to men who are deficient in it, but this treatment is not recommended for any man with prostate problems, since it can exacerbate them and can add to the growth of an early prostate cancer.

None of the preceding treatments represents a cure for impotence nor an ideal means of dealing with every man who has the problem; most of them are still experimental, and early findings indicate that each treatment only helps some men.

PENILE PROSTHESES

Since the 1970s, it has been possible for surgeons to implant a solid or inflatable object in the penis to permit a satisfactory erection. A number of different companies manufacture these penile prostheses, which fall into specific categories: rigid and semirigid types; and those with inflatable, hydraulic, or spring devices. Some urologists prefer one particular type, but many are experienced in implanting several types and so are able to offer a choice to their patients.

The manufacturers of prostheses offer illustrated brochures describing their devices, as well as lists of local urologists who have had a great deal of experience implanting them. These manufacturers are listed in appendix 4.

The Small-Carrion Penile Prosthesis, developed by Dr. Michael P. Small and Dr. Herman M. Carrion of the University of Miami School of Medicine, was the first modern prosthesis. Consisting of silicone tubes filled with spongy material, it is surgically inserted into the penis and provides the man with a semirigid penis. It enables him to have satisfactory intercourse, but because it maintains a permanent erection, some men may find it awkward or embarrassing in some situations.

The Flexi-Rod Penile Implant, a later development, is similar to the Small-Carrion, but it is made with flexible silicone rods that are hinged for better concealment, enabling the penis to hang more naturally. The prosthesis is not noticeable when a man is dressed, even in slimline clothes. This prosthesis permits satisfactory intercourse, but achieving penetration with it may be a little more difficult than with the Small-Carrion.

Other prostheses that produce a permanent erection

may be reinforced with metal. Some are malleable or positional, so that they can be positioned close to the body during everyday activities.

Inflatable prostheses consist of hollow cylinders implanted in the penis and filled with fluid by means of a silicone rubber pump placed under the scrotum. Based on a simple procedure using a cylinder, pump, reservoir, and interconnecting tubes, it is all concealed under the skin and cannot be seen from the outside. The reservoir filled with fluid is placed under the abdominal muscles. When the man wants an erection he squeezes the pump, which transfers fluid to the cylinders in the penis, mimicking the way the penis normally fills with blood during an erection. To return the penis to a flaccid position, the man releases the valve on the pump, and the fluid returns to the reservoir.

Self-contained hydraulic prostheses allow the man's genitals to retain a natural-looking appearance; the reservoir and activation devices are contained within the cylinders in the penis. Some do not require any fluid. With one simple motion, the man usually squeezes the inflation pump in the head of the penis to produce an erection, later compressing the deflation site behind the head of the penis to return the penis to a flaccid state.

Solid-rod, hinged, and malleable models are more reasonably priced and less complicated than inflatable and hydraulic ones. All afford impotent men several options for achieving erections. Mechanical failure or malfunction can occur in any type of prosthesis; for this reason a urologist may recommend that the patient choose one that has had a great deal of testing. Deciding which one— if any—to have implanted requires the patient and his urologist to consider many factors: comfort, appearance, concealment, ease of use, and cost.

The patient and the urologist must also discuss

whether the patient is a good candidate for this surgery. Implantation is done in the hospital on either an in-patient or out-patient basis. The surgical procedure is performed through a single incision, which may be made in the lower abdomen near the base of the penis, at the junction where the penis joins the scrotum, or on the shaft of the penis.

As with any surgery, a recovery period is involved. Some pain will be felt for a few weeks following surgery, and very occasionally, an infection may develop. About four to six weeks after implantation, a man can begin to have intercourse. In many instances, he will be able to have orgasms, to ejaculate, and even to father children.

No man should consider implantation of a penile prosthesis without fully exploring his feelings about sexual functioning, his reason for wanting the surgery, and his expectation of what this will mean in his life. If he has a wife or regular partner, the decision should be a joint one. Frequently, a man decides he wants a penile implant to please his partner, only to find out later that the partner would not have concurred in this decision if consulted about it prior to surgery. Some urologists refer any patient contemplating this surgery to a competent sexual counselor prior to (and even after) surgery.

Both partners need to be sure that the man is doing this because he really wants to—not just because it is available. The prosthetic implantation procedure involves surgery and a recovery period, and an occasional (albeit infrequent) complication. A man should ask himself, "Is it worth it?" A couple must also decide whether their inability to engage in intercourse is the only reason they are choosing the prosthesis. A penile prosthesis will *not* solve problems that involve in-laws, money, children, or step-children. Finally, a man without a regular partner needs to consider whether a decision such as this will really make important changes in his life.

For many men who are either having difficulty or are unable to obtain an erection sufficient for penetration, prosthesis is not the answer. For them, loving and caring and sexuality do not depend on sexual intercourse; and they and their partners often decide against a penile prosthesis implant.

NONSURGICAL DEVICES

External vacuum constriction devices are an alternative to surgery. In these devices, a donut-shaped cylinder is placed over a flaccid penis; a pump, connected to the cylinder by means of a tube, is then activated, drawing air from the cylinder either automatically or by mouth. This creates a vacuum inside the cylinder, constricting the cylinder and increasing the amount of blood entering the penile vascular system. The vacuum is then released, and the cylinder slides off the penis, allowing intercourse to begin. This system is completely visible to the partner during operation, which to many men is a decided disadvantage.

External vacuum constriction devices are available to patients only with a prescription from a physician. Like the manufacturers of penile prostheses, the makers of these devices offer descriptive information to potential users and can also refer them to physicians who are familiar with the system. These manufacturers are listed in appendix 4.

People who view sexuality as a shared mutual experience—one that provides both partners with emotional and physical satisfaction, without any specific goal in mind—find great pleasure in life. Unfortunately, their grown children, the media, and some physicians tend to look at older couples with amusement or even disdain when they see them showing signs of anything more than mild affection. But most doctors and counselors who treat people of all ages recognize that sexuality and sexual desire can last a lifetime and that this is the norm rather than the exception.

This book was not intended to provide a "cookbook" approach to achieving sexual success after a prostatectomy or at any particular age or stage of life, but it was meant to convey the profound conviction that it is never too late to enjoy sexual activity. Of course, physiological changes occur with aging, with surgery, and with various treatments, but they need not diminish the pleasure people can take in their sexuality.

Appendix 1

WHEN TO SEE A UROLOGIST

Any of the following problems *may* be related to the prostate. If they do not respond to treatment recommended by the patient's personal physician, he should see a urologist.

- Frequent or urgent need to urinate, including during the night
- Discomfort or pain during urination
- Inability to urinate
- Sensation of incomplete emptying of the bladder
- Pain in the pelvic or rectal area
- Hesitancy to begin to urinate
- Diminution of caliber and force of the urinary stream
- Inability to abruptly stop urination—instead, continuing to dribble
- Blood in urine
- Nausea, dizziness, or unusual sleepiness—sometimes the result of "silent prostatism"

- Appendix 2 -

QUESTIONS TO ASK THE UROLOGIST

Every man with a problem relating to his prostate is different, so some of these questions may not be relevant in a particular case. In addition, every man's physical response to his condition and treatment is different, so the urologist may not be able to answer all of these questions precisely. But the questions will help the patient get a better understanding of his problem, and the answers will provide him with important information. For all prostate problems:

- What do you call the condition I have?
- Is this something that is likely to clear up quickly with treatment, or should I be prepared for a slow recovery?
- How often will I need checkups? Will there be tests? What kind?
- What are the risks of the surgical procedure or other treatment you are recommending?
- What are the risks of *not* having the surgery (or other recommended treatment)?

- What tests will I have before surgery? after surgery?
- Will I have to be hospitalized, or can surgery be performed in the doctor's office or in the hospital on an out-patient basis?
- How long will I be in the hospital for surgery?
- When will I be able to return to everyday activities and to resume sexual relations?
- If I am unable to resume sexual relations—that is, if I am left impotent—what do you suggest? Can you advise me or send me to someone who is an expert in this area?

If the problem is cancer of the prostate:

- Is there a choice between surgery and radiotherapy?
- If I have surgery, what kind will it be? Will it affect my ability to have sex? Do you do the new nerve-sparing surgery?
- If I have radiotherapy, what type will I get— internal? external? Will it affect my ability to have sex?
- Will I need to be hospitalized for radiotherapy? If so, for how long?
- Will I be taking medication? What kind?
- How often and for how long will I need to return for checkups relating to this cancer?
- Will you be scheduling regular tests? What kind?
- What will those tests tell us?
- What are the particular signs of problems that I should be alert for?

Appendix 3

COMPLICATING DRUGS

The following drugs can interfere with prostate conditions or cause impotence:

- Antidepressants
- Tranquilizers
- Antihistamines
- Cough medicines
- Nose sprays
- Sleeping pills
- Heart, hypertension, and ulcer medications
- Alcohol
- Anabolic steroids

- Appendix 4 -

REFERENCE GUIDE TO
FURTHER INFORMATION

FINDING A UROLOGIST

The patient's personal physician or local hospital should be able to recommend a urologist to him. Alternatively, he may call his local medical society and ask for a referral. Most medical societies give three names in response to such requests. The *Directory of Medical Specialists* lists all physicians who are American Board Certified Specialists. A new directory is issued every two years. Many branch libraries have the book, or the librarian can suggest where to find it. Urologists are listed (by community) in the section entitled "Urologists." The credentials or affiliations of any Board Certified physician can be checked by consulting the alphabetical index of the directory.

Most states have a medical directory of all state-licensed physicians; this directory is usually available in local libraries. The American Medical Association (AMA) also publishes a directory of physicians in the United States. These books are good sources of information on physicians.

INFORMATION FOR CANCER PATIENTS AND THEIR FAMILIES

The National Cancer Institute (NCI) supports cancer research throughout the country and also conducts its own research. Of special interest and extreme usefulness to cancer patients and their families is the NCI's information and referral service, the Cancer Information Service (CIS) of the National Cancer Institute. Toll-free phone numbers for the CIS are as follows:

> In the continental United States and Puerto Rico: (800)4-CANCER
> In Hawaii: (808)524-1234 (local in Oahu; from neighboring islands, call collect)

Calling the CIS number connects the caller with the CIS regional office serving his area. That office can provide accurate, personalized answers to all cancer-related questions and can identify various community agencies and services available, including the name and location of the medical library nearest to the caller's home. Upon request, the office will point out the closest Comprehensive Cancer Center and tell where any experimental programs for prostate cancer are being conducted. The CIS office can also help callers find a personal physician.

Spanish-speaking staff members are available to callers from the following areas (daytime hours only): California, Florida, Georgia, Illinois, New Jersey, New York City, and Texas.

NCI's national mailing address is as follows:

Office of Cancer Communications
National Cancer Institute (NCI)
National Institutes of Health
Building 31, Room 1018A
Bethesda, MD 20014

147

Upon request, NCI will send a list identifying written materials available on cancer (in general), on prostate cancer, or on any other specified cancer.

ACS's national mailing address and phone number are as follows:

American Cancer Society (ACS)
National Headquarters
4 West 35th Street
New York, NY 10001
(212)736-3030

Besides funding research, the American Cancer Society sponsors several patient-support programs such I Can Cope (an educational program for patients and families) and CanSurmount (a patient-to-patient support service). Many local ACS divisions and units can help cancer patients with transportation (either through financial aid or through a program called Road to Recovery), and some offer care in the home.

Local American Cancer Society divisions and units are listed in the telephone directory. These offices can provide information about locally available services, as well as various written materials.

The Canadian Cancer Society's national mailing address and phone number are as follows:

The Canadian Cancer Society
130 Bloor Street West, suite 1001
Toronto, Ontario, Canada M58 2V7
(416)961-7223

It offers many of the same services as the American Cancer Society and maintains divisions in every province. The telephone directory lists the nearest division office.

FINDING A PAIN SPECIALIST

Calling the CIS toll-free number is the easiest way to find the name of the nearest university- or hospital-based pain clinic. If this pain clinic is too far away to allow treatment there, a patient's personal physician can contact the clinic or it can recommend a pain specialist near the patient's home. The county medical society may also be able to give the patient a referral.

INFORMATION AND REFERRALS ON SEXUAL FUNCTIONING, IMPOTENCE, OR URINARY INCONTINENCE

The American Association of Sex Educators,
   Counselors and Therapists
11 Dupont Circle, N.W.
Suite 220
Washington, DC 20036
(202)462-1171

This organization certifies sex counselor-therapists and can provide a list of such professionals in the patient's area.

SIECUS (Sex Information and Education Council of the
   United States)
80 Fifth Avenue
New York, NY 10011

This group provides information on books, periodicals, and organizations involved with the subjects of sexuality and illness. For $1 (and a stamped, self-addressed #10 envelope), SIECUS will send this list, entitled *Sexuality and Disability: A Bibliography of Resources Available for Purchase*.

Impotence Institute International and Impotence Institute of America
Impotents Anonymous (IA) [for impotent men] and
I-ANON [for partners of impotent men]
119 South Ruth Street
Maryville, TN 37801-5746
(615)983-6064

This organization was founded in 1983 to inform and educate the general public about the causes and treatment of impotence and to conduct and sponsor programs for carrying out these purposes. The organization has an excellent newsletter and other publications. A videotape entitled *Impotence: Help and Hope* is also available. Meetings of IA and I-ANON, modeled after the fellowship programs of Alcoholics Anonymous, are held nationwide. Chapters have lay coordinators, but urologists also play an important role in meetings. Further information is available from the national headquarters. Enclose a self-addressed, stamped envelope.

ROMP (Recovery of Male Potency)
Grace Hospital
18700 Mayers Road
Detroit, MI 48235
(800)TEL-ROMP [or (800)835-7667]
in Michigan: (313)966-3219

The chapters of this organization are all hospital-based and serve as information and referral services, as well as offering emotional support. People calling the organization's phone number will speak with a nurse, who can refer them to appropriate local sources of help. ROMP publishes a newsletter and other informational material.

The Simon Foundation
Box 835 Z
Wilmette, IL 60091
(800)237-4666

This organization serves as an information and referral service to individuals suffering from incontinence. It offers a newsletter and a number of publications.

MANUFACTURERS OF PENILE PROSTHESES AND NONSURGICAL DEVICES

The following manufacturers will send patients information on these devices, as well as a list of implanting surgeons in their area:

Impotence Information Center
American Medical Systems
P.O. Box 9
Minneapolis, MN 55460
(800)328-3881

Surgitek/Medical Engineering Corporation
3037 Mount Pleasant Street
Racine, WI 53404
(800)558-4321
in Wisconsin: (414)639-7205

Dacomed Corporation
1701 East 79th Street
Minneapolis, MN 55425
(800)328-1103

Mentor Corporation
600 Pine Avenue
Goleta, CA 93117
(800)235-5731

Osborn Medical Systems
P.O. Box 1478
1246 Jones Street
Augusta, GA 30903
(800)438-8592 (outside Georgia)
(800)334-2757 (in Georgia)
(800)356-4676 (in Canada)

Response/KSI, Inc.
889 South Matlack Street
West Chester, PA 19382
(800)444-5748

GLOSSARY

abscess
: An accumulation of pus, often resulting in swelling, fever, and pain.

acute
: Rapidly developing, quick, sudden.

ampulla
: A small dilation in a canal or duct.

androgens
: Hormones that encourage the development and maintenance of male sex characteristics. Testosterone is an androgen. Absence of androgens will usually cause the prostate to shrink.

anesthetic
: A substance that causes loss of sensation in all or part of the body. General anesthetic causes lack of consciousness and sensation. Local anesthetic causes only lack of sensation.

antihistamine
: Any of a group of drugs used to relieve the symptoms of allergies and colds. Antihistamines work by neutralizing the effects of histamine, an active substance in allergic reactions.

antihormones
: Drugs that work to block hormones that stimulate cancer growth.

anus
: The opening found at the end of the digestive tract, through which waste products are excreted.

artery   A large blood vessel that carries blood from heart to tissues.

aspiration   The removal by suction of air, fluid, or tissue from an area in the body.

atrophy   The emaciation, shrinking, or wasting of tissues, organs, or the entire body for any of a number of possible causes. For example, a man's testes will atrophy (although the scrotum will remain intact) if he is deprived of male hormones or given female hormones.

bacteria   A broad class of one-celled microorganisms, some of which must live and feed off other living things. Many (but not all) bacteria are capable of causing disease.

benign   Characteristic of a mild illness or a nonmalignant growth. A benign (or nonmalignant) tumor is one that does not invade and destroy neighboring normal tissue.

benign prostatic hypertrophy (BPH)   The enlargement or growth of the glandular tissue within the prostatic capsule. BPH does not spread or attack other tissue or cells, but it can push the prostate outward, thus narrowing the bladder outlet.

bilateral   Possessing or related to two sides.

154

biopsy
A procedure whereby tissue is removed from living patients so that it can be further studied, to aid the physician in making a medical diagnosis.

bladder
In medical usage, the urinary bladder—an elastic sac that serves to store urine before it is excreted from the body.

blood acid phosphatase level
The relative amount of phosphatase in blood. Phosphatase is an enzyme found in almost all tissues, body fluids, and cells. An increase of acid phosphatase in the blood may indicate cancer of the prostate, or some other disease.

blood alkaline level
The relative amount of substances capable of neutralizing acids in blood. These alkaline substances play an important role in maintaining normal functioning of the body.

blood cells
Cells that, together with plasma, make up blood. They are manufactured in the bone marrow and include red blood cells, white blood cells, and platelets.

blood count
Calculation of the number of red cells, white cells, and platelets in a given sample of blood. Taking a blood count aids in the diagnosis of a disease or deficiency.

body imaging　Any examination technique that gives a picture of the body's interior (for example, x-rays, nuclear scans, CAT scans, ultrasound, and NMR).

boggy　Soft, spongy, and swollen.

bone marrow　The soft, spongelike material found inside the cavities of bones. It is here that red blood cells, white blood cells, and platelets are made.

bone scan　A picture of the bones obtained by first injecting the patient with a radioactive chemical that travels to the areas around the bone, thus highlighting any bone injury, repair, or destruction. The bone scan is an extremely sensitive test, particularly useful in the diagnosis of prostate cancer that may have metastasized to the bones.

bone survey　A complete series of x-rays of the skeletal system. This survey is used as a diagnostic aid in detecting cancer.

BPH　*See* BENIGN PROSTATIC HYPERTROPHY.

cancer　The uncontrolled growth of abnormal cells. Also called *malignant neoplasm* or *malignancy*.

Candida albicans　A species of yeastlike fungus that usually causes infection of the throat, vagina, and gastrointestinal tract. If left unchecked, it can sometimes lead to more serious disease.

cardiovascular Relating to circulation, to the heart, and to blood vessels.

castration In men, the removal of testicles by surgery, or the suppression of male hormones by administration of female hormones.

catheter A hollow, flexible tube designed to be passed through the urethra into the bladder in order to drain urine.

CAT scan *See* TOMOGRAPHY.

cauterization The burning or scarring of skin or tissue by the use of heat, chemicals, or instruments. Usually done to destroy abnormal tissue.

chemotherapy Treatment of illness by drugs or medication that can reach all parts of the body; most often used to describe the treatment of cancer by drugs that can interfere with cancer-cell growth and destroy cancer cells.

chronic Continuous or of long duration. Certain diseases are chronic in that they slowly progress and/or continue for long periods of time.

coitus Sexual intercourse.

coitus interruptus Conscious withdrawal of the penis during intercourse prior to ejaculation and/or orgasm.

coitus prolongus Conscious postponement of ejaculation and/or orgasm during intercourse.

157

complete blood count (CBC)	*See* BLOOD COUNT.
computerized tomography	*See* TOMOGRAPHY.
congestion	Swelling due to the presence of increased blood in blood vessels or tissues.
congestive prostatitis	A noninfectious form of prostatitis that may be caused by stress, chronic vibration, sexual habits, or other social factors or may be residual after infection.
contraceptive	Any drug, device, or method designed to prevent pregnancy.
contrast medium	A dye injected or gradually flowed into a vein to highlight internal structures for visualization through x-rays and other body-imaging techniques.
Cowper's glands (or bulbourethral glands)	Two glands located on either side of the male urethra. They produce a secretion that becomes part of the seminal fluid.
cryosurgery	Surgery that makes use of an extremely low-temperature probe.
cystoscope	A lighted instrument that is passed through the urethra and into the bladder for examination of the bladder interior.

cystostomy   An opening in urinary bladder with the external opening on the lower abdomen.

–ectomy   A suffix meaning "surgical removal" (of the body part specified in the preceding part of the word, as in *prostatectomy*).

epididymitis   Inflammation of the epididymis.

erection   The enlargement and stiffening of the penis when it becomes filled with blood as a result of sexual stimulation.

estrogens   A general name for female sex hormones made in the ovaries. Although each hormone has a slightly different function, they are closely related and are usually referred to collectively as *estrogen*. Estrogen is responsible for the development of reproductive organs and secondary sex characteristics of women. Synthetic estrogens are used in the treatment of prostatic cancer and in many treatments for conditions in women.

excision   Surgical removal of tissue or a body part.

excretion   The process whereby undigested food and waste products are eliminated from the body.

external radiation   Radiation emitted by a machine directed toward the diseased part of the body.

fascia	A band or sheet of tissue that covers the muscles and various organs of the body, below the skin.
fertile	Capable of conceiving and bearing children.
fiber optics	A branch of optics that makes use of flexible tubelike instruments containing glass or plastic fibers capable of transmitting and bending light and reflecting a magnified image. Instruments of this type can be inserted into the body to make visible otherwise inaccessible areas of the body.
foreskin (or prepuce)	The free fold of skin that covers, more or less completely, the head of the penis. The foreskin is partially or totally removed in circumcision.
genitals (or genitalia)	The male and female reproductive organs, both internal and external.
gland	An organ that selectively removes material from the bloodstream and converts it into a new substance, which may be recirculated through the bloodstream for a specific function or may be excreted.
glans	An acorn-shaped structure: (male) the *glans penis* refers to the tip of the penis; (female) the *glans clitoridis* refers to the small mass of erectile tissue at the tip of the clitoris.
gynecologist	A physician who specializes in diseases, reproductive physiology, and endocrinology of women.

gynecomastia	Excessive enlargement and development of breasts in men.
hematologist	A physician who specializes in problems of the blood and bone marrow.
hematuria	Any condition in which the urine contains blood or red blood cells.
hemospermia	Presence of blood in the seminal fluid.
hormone	A chemical product formed in one part of the body (usually in endocrine glands) that is carried in the blood to other parts. When hormones are secreted into body fluids, they have a specific effect on other organs.
hormonotherapy	The treatment of cancer with hormones, usually in conjunction with other methods such as surgery or chemotherapy.
impotence	Inability of a man to achieve and maintain an erection sufficient for penetration.
incontinence	Inability to prevent discharge of urine or feces.
infection	Usually, the invasion and multiplication of certain diseases caused by microorganisms.
infectious prostatitis	A form of prostatitis caused by an invasion of the prostate by bacteria, yeast, viruses, or other microorganisms.

inflammation	A condition resulting from injury, infection, or irritation. The common signs of inflammation are redness, heat, swelling, and pain.
instill	To put in, in a measured volume.
internal radiation	Radiation emitted by a radioactive substance that has been implanted in the body close to the area that requires radiotherapy.
intracavitary radiation	Radiation emitted from a radioactive source that has been implanted in a body cavity, such as the prostate.
intravenous pyelogram (IVP)	A series of x-ray pictures taken after the intravenous injection of dye into the patient's bloodstream. These x-ray pictures outline the urinary bladder, ureters, and kidneys. The dye is then excreted by the kidneys. This technique is also referred to as *intravenous urography*.
irritative prostatitis	*See* PROSTATODYNIA.
kidneys	Two bean-shaped organs located on each side of the spinal column. Blood passes through them, and the impurities that are removed there dissolve and form urine.
laser	An acronym for *Light Amplification by Stimulated Emission of Radiation*. A laser beam is an extremely concentrated source of light that gives off so much heat that it can destroy anything in its path.

162

lesion	A mass of cells that may be solid, semisolid (cystic), inflammatory, benign, or malignant. The term *lesion* also applies to a lump or abscess.
libido	Conscious or unconscious sexual desire.
localized	Remaining at the site of origin (referring to cancer cells).
lymph	A clear, transparent, watery, sometimes faintly yellowish liquid containing white blood cells and some red blood cells. It travels through the lymph system, removing bacteria from tissues, transporting fat from intestines, and supplying lymphocytes to the blood.
lymphangio-gram, pedal	A diagnostic test used to inspect lymph glands. Dye is injected between the first and second and the second and third toes of each foot, in order to stain the lymphatic vessels.
lymphatic system	The interconnected circulatory system of spaces and vessels that carry lymph throughout the body.
lymph nodes (or lymph glands)	Structures throughout the body that contain lymph. They also act as a defense system, triggering an immune response to cancer as well as to bacteria.
magnetic resonance imaging (MRI)	A diagnostic technique that produces a body-section image and can detect dead or degenerating cells, blockage of blood flow, and cancer.

malignant   Cancerous.

malignant tumor   A growth of cancer cells.

masturbation   The stimulation or manipulation of one's own or another's genital organs for sexual gratification.

medical history   A patient's record of past illness, operations, accidents, and other relevant experiences of the patient. A medical history may also include information about the patient's family and forebears.

metabolism   All physical and chemical processes involved in the maintenance of life and producing tissue change. Basically, these processes are of two types: those that break down larger particles into smaller ones, thereby producing usable energy; and those that convert smaller particles into larger ones, thereby storing energy.

metastasis   The shifting, spread, or colonization of an original cancerous tumor to another part of the body. It is usually transported through the bloodstream or the lymph system.

metastatic lesion   A small patch of malignant tissue (or tumor) that has spread from the original site of cancer, however remote.

microscopic   Too small to be visible to the naked eye, but large enough to be visible under a microscope.

neoplasm	A tumor or abnormal new growth or swelling of tissue. It can be either benign or malignant.
nephritis	Acute or chronic inflammation of the kidneys.
nocturia	The urge or need to urinate at night.
nocturnal emission	A discharge of seminal fluid during sleep. It may be the result of erotic dreams, or simply a natural way to rid the body of accumulated sperm and secretions. Often referred to as a *wet dream*.
nodule	A small mass of tissue or a tumor, generally malignant.
noninfectious prostatitis	*See* CONGESTIVE PROSTATITIS; PROSTATODYNIA.
nuclear scan	A diagnostic test that makes use of a small amount of one or more radioactive trace compounds.
oncologist	A physician specifically trained to treat neoplasms or tumors.
oncology	The study and treatment of neoplasms and tumors.
orchiectomy (or orchidectomy)	The surgical removal of one or both testicles. When an orchiectomy is performed for cancer of the prostate, the scrotum is left intact.

orgasm	The climax of the sexual act, usually accompanied by muscular contractions, release of tension, and pleasurable sensation. In men, orgasm is usually (but not always) accompanied by ejaculation. Orgasm may occur without erection.
palliative treatment	Treatment that is not aimed at cure, but at making a patient feel better by relieving symptoms, pain, or discomfort from a disease.
palpation	A technique in which the physician uses hands (rather than instruments) to examine organs to assess their texture, size, consistency, and location.
pathology	The branch of medicine that deals with the results of disease, particularly as seen in cell, organ, and tissue changes.
pelvis	The lower part of the body (excluding the legs), formed by the two hip bones and the lower portion of vertebral column, and constituting the lowest part of the trunk.
penis	The male organ, used for urinary excretions and for sexual intercourse.
perineal prostatectomy	The removal of all or part of the prostate gland through an incision in the perineum—the area between the anal opening and the scrotum.
peritoneum	The closed, membranous sac that covers the entire abdominal wall of the body.

pituitary gland	An endocrine gland located at the base of the brain. It produces hormones that regulate the secretions of other endocrine glands.
potency	The ability of a man to achieve and maintain an erection sufficient for penetration.
prepuce	*See* FORESKIN.
prognosis	The doctor's forecast of the probable outcome of a disease.
prostate	The male gland that surrounds the urethra. It secretes a fluid that forms part of semen.
prostatectomy	Surgical removal of all or part of the prostate gland. The three types performed are transurethral resection, retropubic and suprapubic.
prostatitis	Acute, chronic, or temporary inflammation of the prostate gland, usually caused by infection, congestion, or irritation.
prostatodynia	A noninfectious prostatitis, whose cause has not been fully established. Stress or irritation may be cause.
prosthesis	An artificial replacement for a missing or nonfunctioning part of the body.
pubis	The area just above external genitals.

radiation   The process of emitting radiant energy in the form of x, light, short radio, ultraviolet, or any other electromagnetic rays from one source or center. In medicine, these rays may be used for treatment or diagnosis.

radiotherapist   A physician who is specially trained in radiotherapy.

radiotherapy   The use of electromagnetic rays (or radiation) in the treatment of disease.

rectum   The end portion of the large intestine, extending from the sigmoid colon to the anal canal.

red blood cells (rbc)   Small, disk-shaped cells that float in blood and contain hemoglobin. They are responsible for the color of the blood, the transport of oxygen to the tissues, and the removal of carbon dioxide from tissues.

red blood count (RBC)   The number of red blood cells per cubic centimeter of blood.

refractory period   The amount of time a man requires after ejaculation and/or orgasm before he is able to achieve a second erection.

resectoscope   An instrument inserted through the urethra during surgery. It is used for the removal of all or part of the prostate gland during a transurethral resection, as well as in other surgical procedures in both men and women.

retrograde ejaculation	The flow of semen backward into the bladder instead of forward through the penis. This phenomenon is a frequent result of prostate surgery.
retropubic prostatectomy	Surgical removal of all or part of the prostate gland through an incision in the lower abdomen, below the navel and slightly above the penis. The bladder is not opened in this procedure.
scan	Computerized picture of an organ or body part, such as the bones, liver, or brain. Radioactive substances are sometimes injected into the patient prior to the scan; these concentrate in the sections of the body to be scanned, thereby improving the image produced.
scrotum	The external sac of skin that contains the testicles.
secretion	A substance that is produced by a cell or group of cells of an organism and stored or utilized by that organism.
seminal fluid (or semen)	A thick, yellowish white fluid that contains spermatozoa. It is a mixture of secretions from the testicles, the seminal vesicles, the prostate gland, and the Cowper's glands.
seminal vesicles	Two folded glandular structures that lie against the lower rear bladder wall. The secretions of the seminal vesicles form part of semen.

septic

Infected.

serum

The fluid portion of the blood, obtained after the blood cells and fibrin clot have been removed.

sexual dysfunction

Inability to achieve sexual relations that result in satisfaction and/or orgasm.

silent prostatism

A condition in which prostatic obstruction exists without symptoms, and can lead to serious kidney damage if not treated.

sitz bath

A regular or therapeutic hot bath in which a person sits down.

sonogram

A computer picture that uses ultrasound (high-frequency sound waves) to examine the position, form, and function of anatomical structures. The vibrations (or waves) are sent through various parts of the body to create a picture of various layers of the body's interior. A sonogram is the record of these ultrasound tests.

sperm (or spermatozoa)

The male sex cell or gamete (composed of a head and a tail), which fertilizes the ovum (female sex cell). Within the sperm is the genetic information from the father that will be transmitted to offspring. Sperm forms part of semen.

sphincter

A ringlike muscle whose relaxation or contraction regulates the amount of substance that can pass through a tube or out of an organ.

staging	Careful evaluation to determine the extent of a patient's disease.
sterile	Unable to produce offspring.
sterilization	The process by which a person is made incapable of producing offspring.
stilbestrol	A synthetic female hormone, frequently given to patients who suffer from cancer of the prostate.
stones (bladder)	Formed by crystallization of urine that remains in bladder or from retained stones from kidneys and ureter.
stricture	A narrowing of a structure or passageway.
suprapubic prostatectomy	The removal of all or part of the prostate gland through an incision made in the skin below the navel and slightly above the pubis in the lower abdomen. The bladder is opened in this procedure.
suture	Surgical stitches bringing together two surfaces.
TENS	*See* TRANSCUTANEOUS ELECTRIC NERVE STIMULATION.
testicles (or testes; singular, testis)	The two male reproductive glands that produce sperm and androgens. They are enclosed in the scrotum.
testosterone	A hormone that encourages the development and maintenance of male sex characteristics.

tomography   A diagnostic technique using computers and x-rays to obtain a highly detailed image of a section of the body being studied.

total prostatectomy   Surgical removal of the entire prostate gland and capsule.

transcutaneous electric nerve stimulation (TENS)   A procedure in which mild electrical stimulation of the skin is used to relieve chronic pain.

transurethral resection (TUR)   Surgical removal of all or part of the prostate gland, accomplished by passing an instrument through the penis and urethra and cutting away tissue in the prostate gland.

tumor   Swelling or enlargement due to abnormal overgrowth of tissue. *Neoplasm* is a term used to refer to tumors that are composed of new and actively growing tissue. Their growth is faster than that of normal tissue and serves no useful purpose. Tumors can be either benign or malignant.

ultrasound   *See* SONOGRAM.

uremia   An excess of urea and other nitrogenous wastes in the blood.

ureter   The long, narrow tube through which urine passes from the kidney to the bladder.

urethra	In men and women, the muscular tube or canal through which urine passes from the bladder and out of the body. In men, seminal fluid as well as urine passes through the urethra.
urine	Fluid that is excreted by the kidneys, stored in the bladder, and expelled through the urethra. Urine consists of 96 percent water and 4 percent dissolved substances.
urologist	A physician who specializes in the diagnosis and treatment of diseases of the male genitourinary tract and the female urinary tract.
vagina	The female genital canal.
varicocele	A varicose condition of the veins of the spermetic cord, causing a benign, boggy tumor of the scrotum.
vas deferens (plural, vasa deferentia)	One of the two tubes attached to the epididymis, extending to the prostatic urethra and looping behind the bladder, where it becomes the ejaculatory duct.
vasectomy	The removal of a part of the vas deferens. Bilateral vasectomy results in sterility.
vein	A blood vessel that carries blood from tissues to the heart and lungs.
venereal disease	A type of disease relating to or resulting from sexual relations. (However, not all diseases related to sex are venereal diseases.

white blood cells (wbc)	Several blood-cell types, containing no hemoglobin, that are active in response to disease, injury, and medication. White blood cells are about one-third larger than red blood cells, and they act against infection.
white blood count (WBC)	The number of white blood cells per cubic centimeter of blood.
workup	The combined results of a medical examination and tests (some of which may be done in a hospital), to arrive at a diagnosis and a complete medical picture of the patient.

RECOMMENDED READING

American Medical Association. *AMA Family Medical Guide*. New York: Random House, 1987.

Benson, Herbert, and Klipper, Miriam Z. *The Relaxation Response*. New York: Avon, 1976.

Berger, Richard E., and Berger, Deborah. *Biopotency: A Guide to Sexual Success*. Emmaus, Pa.: Rodale Press, 1987.

Brecher, Edward M. *Love, Sex and Aging: A Consumer Union Report*. New York: Consumer Union, 1986.

Bricklin, Mark. *Rodale's Encyclopedia of Natural Home Remedies*. Emmaus, Pa.: Rodale Press, 1982.

Brody, Jane. *Jane Brody's Nutrition Book*. New York: Bantam, 1987.

———. *Jane Brody's Good Food Book*. New York: Bantam, 1987.

———. *Jane Brody's The New York Times Guide to Personal Health*. New York: Avon, 1983.

Brooks, Marvin, M.D., and Brooks, Sally West. *How to Avoid and Overcome Impotence*. New York: Doubleday, 1981.

———. *The Lifelong Lover*. New York: Doubleday, 1985.

Butler, Robert, M.D., and Lewis, Myrna, A.C.S.W. *Midlife Love Life*. New York: Harper & Row, 1988.

Carrera, Michael. *Sex: The Facts, the Acts and Your Feelings*. New York: Crown, 1981.

Columbia University College of Physicians and Surgeons. *The Columbia University College of Physicians and Surgeons Complete Home Medical Guide*. New York: Crown, 1985.

Comfort, Alex, M.D. *The Joy of Sex*. New York: Fireside/ Simon & Schuster, 1976.

Covell, Mara Brand. *The Home Alternative to Hospitals and Nursing Homes*. New York: Rawson, 1983.

Freese, Arthur S., and Glabman, Sheldon. *Your Kidneys, Their Care and Their Cure: A Modern Miracle of Medicine*. New York: E. P. Dutton, 1976.

Gartley, Cheryle B., ed. *Managing Incontinence*. Ottawa, Ill.: Jameson Books, 1985.

Hogue, Kathleen; Jensen, Cheryl, and Urban, Kathleen Mc-Clurg. *A Complete Guide to Health Insurance*. New York: Walker, 1988.

Klimann, Peter R., M.D., and Mills, Katherine S. *All About Sex Therapy*. New York: Plenum Press, 1983.

Long, James W. *The Essential Guide to Prescription Drugs*. New York: Harper & Row, 1987.

Morra, Marion, and Potts, Eva. *Choices: Realistic Alternatives in Cancer Treatment*, rev. ed. New York: Avon, 1987.

Moskowitz, Mark, and Osband, Michael E. *The Complete Book of Medical Tests: A Lifetime Guide for You and Your Family*. New York: Norton, 1984.

Mylander, Maureen. *The Healthy Male: A Comprehensive Health Guide for Men*. Boston: Little, Brown, 1987.

Nierenberg, Judith, R.N., and Janovic, Florence. *The Hospital Experience*. New York: Berkley, 1985.

Pinckney, Cathey, and Pinckney, Edward R., M.D. *The Patient's Guide to Medical Tests*, 3d ed. New York: Facts on File, 1986.

Rosenthal, Saul, M.D., *Sex Over Forty*. Los Angeles: J. P. Tarcher, 1987 (distrib. by New York: St. Martins).

Siegel, Mary-Ellen. *The Cancer Patient's Handbook*. New York: Walker, 1986.

Silber, Sherman, M.D. *The Male: From Infancy to Old Age*. New York: Scribners, 1982.

Simon, Gilbert, and Silverman, Harold. *The Pill Book*, 3d ed. New York: Bantam, 1986.

Starr, Bernard D., and Weiner, Marcella Bakur. *The Starr-Weiner Report on Sex and Sexuality in The Mature Years.* New York: McGraw-Hill, 1982.

Weg, Ruth B., ed. *Sexuality in the Later Years: Roles and Behavior.* Orlando, Fla.: Academic Press, 1983.

Westheimer, Ruth. *Dr. Ruth's Guide to Good Sex.* New York: Warner, 1984.

————. *Dr. Ruth's Guide for Married Lovers.* New York: Warner, 1987.

In addition: "Sex Over Forty," a newsletter directed to mature adults is available by subscription. Write: S/40, P.O. Box 1600, Chapel Hill, N.C. 27515 or call 1-800-334-5474 for information and rates.

INDEX

179